W9-BZM-838

Understanding Mental Retardation

Understanding Health and Sickness Series
Miriam Bloom, Ph.D.
General Editor

Understanding Mental Retardation

Patricia Ainsworth, M.D., FAPA
Pamela Baker, Ph.D., FAAMR

University Press of Mississippi
Jackson

www.upress.state.ms.us

The University Press of Mississippi is a member of the Association of
American University Presses.

Copyright © 2004 by University Press of Mississippi
All rights reserved
Manufactured in the United States of America

12 11 10 09 08 07 06 05 04 4 3 2 1
∞
Library of Congress Cataloging-in-Publication Data

Ainsworth, Patricia, M.D.
  Understanding mental retardation / Patricia Ainsworth, Pamela Baker.
    p. cm. — (Understanding health and sickness series)
  Includes bibliographical references and index.
  ISBN 1-57806-646-8 (cloth : alk. paper) — ISBN 1-57806-647-6 (pbk. :
alk paper)
  1. Mental retardation. I. Baker, Pamela C., 1950– II. Title. III. Series.
  RC570.A43 2004
  616.85'88—dc22   2003025098

British Library Cataloging-in-Publication Data available

Contents

Introduction

The true mark of a civilized society may be the manner in which it deals with members who are unlike others. Defining or categorizing people is our mechanism for understanding and coping with variance. In doing so, we often lose sight of our greater similarities. This generalization is especially true of the group of individuals currently described as "mentally retarded."

The term mental retardation is familiar to most Americans, but the term and its variants (mentally retarded, retardation, retarded, mentally deficient, etc.) are not universally accepted; many believe that it stigmatizes and promotes a negative image. While mental retardation is the term commonly used in the United States, this set of conditions is referred to as "intellectual disability" in the British Commonwealth and by the International Society for the Scientific Study of Intellectual Disabilities. In their report "Use of the Term 'Mental Retardation': Language, Image and Public Education" (June 14, 2002), Stephen R. Schroeder of the University of Kansas and his colleagues note that many parents and other advocates in the U.S. prefer the term "learning disability," believing that it is less stigmatizing. The report points to the California experience, where the term mental retardation was discouraged in the school system while the term learning disability was advocated. This led to a 200% increase in the identification of children with learning disabilities and a decrease in the diagnosis of mental retardation. In some California school systems the term mental retardation is banned altogether.

The Schroeder report also points out that many advocates and professionals prefer the use of more precise descriptors such as Down syndrome or fragile X syndrome to the generic term mental retardation. Unfortunately, there are still many people with mental retardation for whom the cause is unknown.

Nearly all leaders in the field favor changing the term mental retardation, but there is no universally agreed-upon alternative. Stephen Taylor, the editor of one of the journals of the American Association on Mental Retardation, held a symposium on the name-change issue in 2002. One contributor held the opinion that most people with mental retardation and their allies "will never be satisfied with any designating term whatsoever. . . . If one is trying to find a term . . . that will finally satisfy those to whom it will be applied, one may as well give up this quest as futile, because there is no such term, and there never will be."

Understanding Mental Retardation uses the common terminology but respectfully acknowledges the very real concerns with regard to terms and stigma.

Mental retardation affects at least 1.4% of the U.S. population, or 2 to 2.5 million people. With appropriate family and societal support, bolstered by reasonable educational and occupational opportunities, 90% of individuals with mental retardation have a good chance for healthy, happy, productive lives. In 1998, over 600,000 children between the ages of 6 and 21 years were classified as having mental retardation although they were in public schools. This estimate did not include children with multiple disabilities or preschool-aged children who may have mental retardation.

Mental retardation cuts across racial, ethnic, educational, cultural, social, religious, and economic backgrounds. Mild mental retardation is slightly more common among males than females but more severe forms of retardation are equally common among both sexes. One in ten U.S. families is directly impacted by mental retardation.

The life expectancy of individuals with retardation is generally correlated with the severity of retardation. The death rate for children and adolescents below 19 years of age who have mild to moderate mental retardation is twice that of their peers. Rates for similarly aged individuals with more severe forms of mental retardation are even higher, approaching 7 to 31 times greater than their peers. Fortunately, with improved medical care and environmental support, the life expectancy of individuals with mental retardation is increasing for those who survive the crucial first year of life.

The concept of retardation is unique in that it does not deal with a specific illness or disease, but with a heterogeneous group of people that share only one trait: below average intellectual and adaptive capacities.

In this book we review the causes of mental retardation, its impact on individuals and families, its different manifestations, current standards of assessment and treatment, issues of prevention and education, and the most recent research.

Chapter 1 discusses the causes of mental retardation, the signs and symptoms of specific forms of mental retardation, and issues of prevention. For the sake of comparison, chapter 2 describes concepts of normal human development while chapter 3 provides historical reference, information about the development of testing for intelligence and adaptive behavior, and definitions of mental retardation and other developmental disabilities.

Chapters 4, 5, and 6 discuss assessment, educational, legislative, and supportive issues important for infants and young children, adolescents, teens, and adults with mental retardation. Chapter 7 discusses the aging adult with mental retardation, continuous learning and recreational opportunities for elder individuals, lifelong support needs, and health care issues relative to long-term care.

Chapter 8 reviews diagnostic and treatment issues involved when individuals with mental retardation also experience other disorders (such as epilepsy and mental illness) that may further compromise their cognitive and adaptive skills. Recent advances in the understanding of the biology of mental retardation are discussed in chapter 9, as well as developments in treatment technology.

In addition, there are four appendixes. Appendix A defines who may benefit from genetic counseling. Appendix B lists the milestones of human development. Appendixes C and D deal with pertinent federal legislation/regulations and available resources, respectively.

Understanding Mental Retardation

1. What Is Mental Retardation and Who Is Affected?

Mental retardation is a syndrome of delayed or disordered brain development evident before age 18 years that results in difficulty learning information and skills needed to adapt quickly and adequately to environmental changes.

Effective prevention of mental retardation is stymied because there are so many different causes. More than one possible cause is suggested in as many as 50% of cases. The causes may include genetic factors, prenatal influence, and environmental factors following birth. For 75% of children with mild symptoms and 30–40% of those with severe symptoms, no specific cause is apparent.

Psychosocial issues have also been implicated in the development of mental retardation. So-called "psychosocial retardation" has been closely linked to an impoverished environment. Indeed, most psychosocial factors act in combination and vary between different lower socioeconomic groups. Prevalence estimates are higher among impoverished individuals and non-Caucasian races; however, the relevance of race to development of mental retardation may be coincidental if non-Caucasians are over-represented in the study group of impoverished people. Isolating any specific impact of poverty is therefore difficult. Further, psychosocial issues in the mental development of a child are subject to disagreement. It is important to remember that the vast majority of individuals living in poverty display normal intellectual function.

Table 1.1 Common Causes of Mental Retardation

Unknown	Largest category
Brain injury	Prenatal and postnatal; ex., cerebral hemorrhage, hypoxia, severe head injury
Infectious	Congenital and postnatal; ex., rubella, meningitis, encephalitis, congenital cytomegalovirus, congenital toxoplasmosis, HIV
Chromosomal abnormalities	Ex., errors in numbers of chromosomes or placement of genes on chromosomes, other defects in chromosomes
Gene abnormalities and inherited metabolic disorders	Ex., galactosemia, Tay-Sachs disease, phenylketonuria, Lesch-Nyhan syndrome, Rett syndrome, tuberous sclerosis
Metabolic	Ex., Reye's syndrome, congenital hypothyroidism, hypoglycemia
Toxic	Ex., intrauterine exposure to alcohol, cocaine, amphetamines, other drugs, methylmercury, lead
Nutritional	Ex., malnutrition
Environmental	Ex., poverty, low socioeconomic status

While mental retardation can be caused by genetic abnormalities or by exposure to noxious conditions (during fetal development or in childhood), the most common known cause of mental retardation is chromosomal abnormalities, of which Down syndrome is the best known. Chromosomal abnormalities may occur in the formation of either of the gametes (egg or sperm) or in the early cell divisions of embryo development. Many authorities believe as many as 40–60% of severe mental retardation can be attributed to such abnormalities.

Perinatal (the time immediately before, during, and shortly after birth) factors account for approximately 11% of severe mental retardation.

Postnatal (the time period from birth through childhood) causes, such as brain injury and severe malnutrition, are responsible for approximately 3–12% of severe retardation. In general, severe retardation is less likely to be inherited. Instead, postnatal environmental factors are suspected—nutrition, maternal health, early childhood health issues, socioeconomic level, access to health care, and exposure to toxic pollutants or chemicals. Identifiable causes are usually multiple and represent less severe insults to the brain.

The Role of Heredity

The genetic template is carried on 46 chromosomes—strands of DNA (deoxyribonucleic acid), each (except for one chromosome) with thousands of genes arranged in a row. Through production of specific proteins, single genes (and more often groups of genes) determine the physical patterns of the human body, including such well-recognized hereditary traits as hair, eye, and skin color as well as stature, body type, and sex. Genes also determine all life functions, such as the efficiency of the liver in clearing toxins and unneeded substances (breakdown products of food and medications, etc.) from the bloodstream, the ability of the pancreas to regulate the use and storage of sugar in the body, the ability of the body to form blood clots at wound sites, and the activities of the brain and central nervous system that we refer to as intelligence, talent, temperament, and athletic ability.

Human chromosomes differ in shape and length, but each human cell (except for the specialized cells of reproduction and red blood cells) contains the chromosomes in pairs—one pair of sex chromosomes and 22 pairs of nonsex chromosomes, called autosomes.

The sex chromosomes are designated by the letters "X" and "Y." Two X chromosomes (usually written as "XX") determine female sex while one chromosome of each type (usually written as "XY") determine male sex. Girls receive one X chromosome from each parent. Boys receive an X chromosome from their mother and a Y chromosome from their father.

The X chromosome also carries non-sex-related genes, and some autosomes also carry genes involved in sex determination. The Y chromosome is primarily a determinant of male sex and carries little additional genetic information.

Transmission of many traits follows patterns of inheritance originally described by Gregor Mendel, the Austrian monk of the mid-nineteenth century who discovered the inheritance of particles in peas and laid the foundation for the modern science of genetics. His description of principles of heredity, known as Mendelian laws of inheritance, focuses on the "phenotype," a term that refers to observable physical characteristics such as stature or eye color or premature graying of the hair. Such physical characteristics reflect individual gene pairs.

The "genotype" describes the genes occupying specific sites on each of the paired chromosomes. Many genes have different forms—for instance, a gene for brown eyes and a gene for blue eyes. Differing forms of the same gene are referred to by geneticists as "alleles." When both genes of a given pair are the same, they are said to be "homozygous." When they differ, they are described as "heterozygous."

Some forms of a gene are more likely to be phenotypically expressed than other forms; that is, the "dominant" gene has greater "penetrance" than the "recessive" gene. The recessive gene is masked when a dominant gene is present and is only apparent when its partner gene is also recessive. The reason seems to be that recessive genes have mutated; that is, they don't make the protein they're supposed to make, while dominant genes produce enough of the protein to make up for the mutation. Thus, for a recessive trait to appear, both genes must be alike. Such is the case with eye-color phenotypes. The gene for brown eyes is "dominant," the gene for blue eyes "recessive." Therefore, individuals with the phenotype of brown eyes may have one of two genotypes for eye color—they may carry two genes for brown eye color (be "homozygous" for the trait) or they may carry one gene for brown eyes and one gene for blue eyes (be "heterozygous" for the trait). Obviously, variations of eye color exist between true brown and true blue—for instance, green or hazel—indicating that all is not as straightforward as it may seem in mendelian inheritance and that "expression" of a dominant gene may be incomplete.

Mendel's laws of inheritance apply to genes on the X chromosomes with a variation stemming from the fact that there is only one X chromosome in normal males and essentially no genes on the Y chromosome to pair with genes on the X chromosome. Furthermore, in 1949, geneticists Barr and Bertram discovered that the cells of normal females contain only one recognizable X chromosome (rather than the expected pair) and one darkly staining mass of condensed DNA, now called the Barr body. Later, geneticist Mary Lyon recognized that the Barr body is the remnant of the missing second X chromosome in females. The Lyon hypothesis proposes that early in development, probably at around the 200–400 cell stage (blastula), one of the two X chromosomes is inactivated (although apparently not all its genes are inactivated) and condensed, forming the Barr body. The selection of the X chromosome to be inactivated is relatively (although not entirely) random, and the same X chromosome is not inactivated in all cells. Thus, beginning at the blastula stage of development in females, there are two different cells lines; one with the maternal X chromosome in place and the paternal one inactivated, and another with the reverse lineage. Normal females are therefore "mosaics" with respect to their X chromosomes.

Further complicating the mendelian laws of inheritance is gene "imprinting," a process by which the gene's ability to express itself is dependent on whether it came from the mother or from the father. In gene imprinting, an as yet unknown process marks the gene of one parent or the other and, in effect, silences or limits its expression. The gene may be marked differently during male versus female germ cell (i.e., sperm vs. egg) formation. In effect, apparently identical genes exhibit dissimilar functions based on whether they came from the father or from the mother. This gene inactivation results in its partner gene (supplied by the other parent) being expressed without respect to the usual issues of dominance and recessiveness of either gene. In other words, a gene that is usually dominant may be inactivated prior to its being transmitted by a parent to a child. When this occurs, the allele transmitted by the other parent will be expressed in the child even if the gene is usually recessive. This process is sometimes referred to as the "parent-of-origin" effect.

Gene imprinting apparently involves a procedure similar to the process that inactivates one of the pair of X chromosomes in females. Gene imprinting on chromosome 15 is present in Prader-Willi syndrome and Angelman syndrome. X-inactivation is present in Rett syndrome. All three of these disorders involve mental retardation and will be discussed below.

The Role of Genetic Disorders in Mental Retardation

Most traits are transmitted with fidelity from one generation to the next. Spontaneous changes (mutations) occasionally occur in genes or chromosomes and may be transmitted to children. These changes may lead to genetic disorders.

More than 500 genetic disorders associated with retardation have been identified. Genetic disorders are generally one of three types: single gene, chromosomal, or multifactorial. Recent advances in genetics, notably by the Human Genome Project, indicate that many disorders formerly classified as single gene or chromosomal in origin are determined by multiple genes on one or more chromosomes.

Single Gene Disorders

Single gene disorders are caused by one mutant gene and are relatively common, occurring in approximately 1 in 100 live births. At least 4,000 to 5,000 known human disorders are caused by single gene abnormalities. In more than 300 disorders, the biochemical abnormality caused by the defective gene has been identified.

Depending on whether the gene in question is located on an autosome or on a sex chromosome, a particular trait may be described as having one of four classic mendelian patterns of inheritance: autosomal dominant, autosomal recessive, X-linked dominant, or X-linked recessive. (As previously noted, the Y chromosome appears to carry few if any active genes except those determining male sex.) As described above, a fifth pattern of inheritance—gene imprinting—also occurs.

While autosomal and X-linked inheritance patterns are based on single gene abnormalities where one gene controls one trait, many traits are transmitted by a combination of genes. These multigenic inheritance patterns are complex and difficult to study, especially since the expression of many of them may be altered by interaction with the environment.

Autosomal dominant inheritance

Children of one parent with an autosomal dominant trait will have a 50% or a 100% chance of inheriting the trait depending, respectively, on whether the affected parent is heterozygous or homozygous for the gene. Male and female children are equally likely to be affected. Neurofibromatosis (also called von Recklinghausen disease) and tuberous sclerosis are examples of single dominant gene disorders that involve mental retardation.

Neurofibromatosis

Neurofibromatosis affects the central nervous system and produces one of the most common forms of mental retardation caused by a single autosomal dominant gene. Up to a third of individuals with neurofibromatosis may have mild retardation. An additional number may have learning disabilities.

In March 2002, Lomas J. Bello and his colleagues described two varieties of the disorder: types 1 and 2, caused by a single mutation on either chromosome 17 or 22, respectively. Type 2 neurofibromatosis usually does not cause skin fibromas or café au lait spots (see table 1.2).

Neurofibromatosis occurs in approximately 1 in 5,000 births. Perhaps half are not inherited but caused by a new mutation.

Table 1.2 Common Signs of Neurofibromatosis

Café-au-lait spots (faded tan birthmarks on the skin)

Neurofibromas (benign tumors caused by abnormal cell migration during embryonic development; includes optic gliomas and acoustic neuromas)

Diffuse freckling

Scoliosis (abnormal curvature of the spine) and other skeletal abnormalities

This is one of the highest mutation rates known for a human disorder.

Tuberous sclerosis

Tuberous sclerosis is characterized by a predisposition to benign tumors in body tissues, especially skin and brain (more than 90% of cases). First described by von Recklinghausen in 1862, "tuberous sclerosis" was-named by Bourneville in 1880 due to the characteristic small benign tumors ("tubers").

With 52.4% of cases thus affected, tuberous sclerosis is second only to neurofibromatosis as a common cause of retardation thought to be produced by a single autosomal dominant gene. Geneticist M. Smith of the University of California at Irvine disputes the single gene theory, believing that the disorder involves multiple genes on multiple chromosomes with a high frequency of new mutations. According to his research, approximately 40% of cases involve chromosome 9 while 56% involve chromosome 16.

Tuberous sclerosis occurs in approximately 1 in 8,000–12,000 live births. The abnormal gene coding for tuberous sclerosis may be inherited but also may occur by spontaneous mutation in 56–86% of cases (OMIM).

Tuberous sclerosis affects all body tissues and, consequently, many body organs—in particular the brain, retina of the eye, skin, kidneys, heart, and lungs (see table 1.3). The so-called "classic triad" of tuberous sclerosis, present in almost 30% of cases, includes mental retardation, epilepsy, and adenoma sebaceum (small, colored nodules on the nose and cheeks).

Mental retardation and seizures in tuberous sclerosis are apparently related to the presence of lesions in the cortex and white matter of the brain. Seizures occur in all affected individuals with retardation and in many without retardation. Cranial X-rays show evidence of calcifications deep inside the

Table 1.3 Common Signs of Tuberous Sclerosis

Adenoma sebaceum (facial angiofibromas—small bright red or brownish nodules that occur in a butterfly distribution on the nose and cheeks—that become apparent between 2 and 5 years of age and are found in over 80% of individuals by late childhood)

Ash-leaf spots (irregular or oval, unpigmented or hypopigmented areas of skin on the arms, trunk, and legs—usually present at birth). When two or more ash-leaf spots are present in an infant, the diagnosis of tuberous sclerosis is strongly suspected.

Shagreen patches (thickened areas of skin usually over the back)

Fibromas inside the mouth, usually occurring under the tongue or on the gums

Retinal lesions (lesions at the edge of the retina of the eye in 50% of individuals; usually do not impair vision)

Cyst-like bone lesions

Sclerotic patches (tuberous lesions scattered throughout the gray matter of the cerebral cortex—visualized by X-ray or brain scans; present at birth, enlarge and calcify with age)

Multiple fibromas (benign tumors in many organs, especially the kidneys, heart, liver, spleen, and lungs)

---

brain in 50% of affected people. CT scans may reveal the deep brain lesions earlier in their development than do X-ray studies.

Physical symptoms may be subtle, often leading to under-diagnosis. Fibrous-angiomatous lesions, present in 83% of individuals with neurofibromatosis, are generally located on the face (but may also be elsewhere) and vary in color from flesh to pink to yellow to brown.

Autosomal recessive inheritance

In autosomal recessive inheritance the mutation is expressed only when both alleles of the gene are present, and requires that both parents pass a recessive gene to the child. The parents may not express the trait themselves if they are not homozygous for the gene but may be heterozygous "carriers." When both parents carry one copy of the same recessive gene, the chance of a child expressing the recessive trait is one in four.

Inborn errors of metabolism represent a group of more than 350 disorders caused by a single genetic defect. Most inborn metabolic errors are a result of an autosomal recessive inheritance pattern because most with an autosomal dominant pattern are lethal and thus not transmitted. Phenylketonuria, homocystinurias, and maple syrup urine disease are examples of inborn metabolic disorders.

Mutations that block a metabolic pathway represent the greatest number of known causes of retardation. The abnormal effects result from a buildup of metabolic products before the block or the lack of a necessary product behind it. Left undiagnosed and untreated, these inborn conditions generally lead to mental retardation. Early diagnosis, treatment, and regular evaluation are keys to reducing the effects of such disorders in affected newborns and infants.

Phenylketonuria

Phenylketonuria (PKU), described in individuals with mental retardation by Ivar Asbjorn Folling in 1934, is the most common and best studied inborn error of metabolism. An infant born with PKU cannot metabolize phenylalanine—an essential amino acid (i.e., one that must be included in the diet)—due to lack of the liver enzyme hepatic phenylalanine hydroxylase. As a result, phenylalanine and its metabolite phenylpyruvic acid build up to toxic levels that can produce brain damage.

PKU can be caused by more than 44 different mutations at the same locus, primarily on chromosome 12, although abnormalities on chromosomes 4 and 11 may produce the syndrome. The disorder occurs in varying degrees of severity. Mild forms occur when the defective gene has limited expression and some normal enzyme is produced; unfortunately, these milder forms of PKU may be missed since phenylalanine levels rise slowly during the first days of life yet still cause mental retardation.

All babies born in the U.S. are routinely screened for PKU. The disorder occurs in approximately 1 in 10,000 live births and is more common in individuals of northern European origin, although cases of PKU have been described in other ethnic groups.

The parents of children with PKU can be treated PKU homozygotes or heterozygous carriers. The child's normal siblings may also be heterozygous carriers. The disorder can be detected in carriers by a phenylalanine tolerance test, a factor that may be important for genetic counseling of family members. (See Appendix A.)

Individuals with untreated PKU are typically hyperactive, erratic and unpredictable in behavior, and difficult to manage. They frequently display temper tantrums and bizarre movements of their bodies and upper extremities with twisting hand mannerisms. Verbal and nonverbal communication is usually severely impaired or nonexistent. Coordination problems, hallucinations, and seizures are common.

Early recognition of PKU can allow dietary intervention with a low phenylalanine diet (in use since 1955). Early intervention significantly improves both behavior and developmental progress, especially if the diet is begun before the child is six months of age. Children who are begun on proper treatment before the age of three months may develop with normal intelligence. For untreated older children and adolescents with PKU, a low phenylalanine diet does not influence the level of mental retardation, but the diet does decrease irritability and abnormal electroencephalogram (i.e., EEG or "brain wave" test) changes. The diet also increases social responsiveness and attention span.

An unforeseen problem has resulted from the success of PKU screening and early treatment measures. Young women with PKU who benefitted from early screening and treatment are now producing children of their own. Many of these women discontinued their low-phenylalanine diet many years prior to producing their children. Because central nervous system damage is not a threat after the early years of development, these women have outgrown the need for the restrictive diet. However, because the phenylalanine levels in their blood remain high, they do expose their developing fetuses to high maternal phenylalanine blood levels that increase the risk of birth defects, including microcephaly (i.e., small head), mental retardation, facial distortion, growth retardation, and congenital heart disease, even if the infant did not inherit PKU.

Homocysteinurias

Homocysteinurias are a group of metabolic disorders of the amino acid methionine. The classic form of the disorder is caused by a gene defect on the long arm of chromosome 21, leading to decreased activity of the enzyme necessary to metabolize homocysteine to cysteine. This results in accumulation of methionine and homocysteine (as well as lack of the metabolic product normally produced) which are excreted in abnormally high concentrations in the urine. Mutations on chromosomes 1 and 5 may also cause the disorder.

People with this disorder tend to exhibit long thin fingers and abnormalities of the lens of their eyes. They frequently have blond hair and reduced skin pigmentation. They may also have a specific body or urine odor (sometimes described as "musty"), eczema, episodic vomiting, and seizures.

Retardation occurs in about half of cases, varying in severity. The mental impairment caused by this classic form of homocysteinuria may be reduced by a methionine-restricted diet supplemented with cysteine. Long-term dietary supplementation of vitamin B_6 can reduce the severity of mental retardation in at least one form of the disorder.

Maple syrup urine disease

Maple syrup urine disease is a third example of an inborn error of amino acid metabolism. The incidence of maple syrup urine disease is estimated to be 1 in 220,000. The disorder may be caused by a mutation on any one of three chromosomes (1, 6, or 19) and is transmitted via an autosomal recessive pattern.

Four clinical variants have been identified: severe (classic), intermittent, intermediate, and thiamine-responsive (Wong, et al. 1972). The classic type (most common) is an acute variant that results in rapid, progressive deterioration of the central nervous system during the first weeks of life. Central nervous system damage can be mitigated by early detection and use of a synthetic diet lacking in branched-chain amino acids. Treatment with long-term thiamine supplementation may also be helpful by improving the stability of a necessary enzyme allowing partial reversal of the block in the metabolic pathway.

The intermittent type results in serious metabolic distortions precipitated by physiological stress, such as minor infections. Episodes can be partially prevented by use of a protein-restricted diet. The intermediate form of the disorder usually does not cause mental retardation. The thiamine-resistant type may be partially reversed by long-term thiamine supplementation, which improves the stability of a necessary enzyme allowing partial reversal of the blocked metabolic pathway.

X-linked dominant inheritance

Genetic transmission may also be sex-linked, primarily X-linked. Because females have two X chromosomes, they may show dominant or recessive inheritance patterns as occurs with autosomal chromosomes. Males will exhibit whichever trait their single X chromosome carries because there is no corresponding allele on the Y chromosome.

X-linked dominant inheritance patterns result when the X chromosome carries a dominant gene. Thus, a woman who is heterozygous for the gene has a 50% chance of passing a trait to each of her daughters (XX) and sons (XY). The woman who is homozygous for the trait will pass the trait to 100% of her children. On the other hand, an affected man will pass his single X chromosome to all his daughters and none of his sons. Thus, his daughters will exhibit the dominant trait while his sons will not.

X-linked recessive inheritance

X-linked recessive inheritance patterns result in traits being expressed more often in males than in females. Women who carry the recessive gene may transmit the gene to their daughters and sons while men can only transmit it to their daughters.

Lesch-Nyhan syndrome

Lesch-Nyhan syndrome is an X-linked recessive condition that can be caused by any one of at least 17 independent mutations. The abnormality produces an inborn error of purine metabolism and occurs in approximately 1 in 100,000 births.

Lesch-Nyhan syndrome causes retardation and severe compulsive self-mutilation. Affected individuals are notorious for their compulsion to bite their lips and fingers, often causing serious physical damage. They also exhibit microcephaly, seizures, choreoathetosis (writhing movements of trunk and extremities), and spasticity.

Disorders Caused by Chromosome Abnormalities

Chromosome-based disorders affect 7 of every 1,000 infants. The disorders are caused by too many or too few chromosomes or by structural abnormalities. An estimated half of all first-trimester miscarriages (i.e., spontaneous abortions) are thought to result from chromosome abnormality. Children born with a chromosome abnormality usually have multiple birth defects and mental retardation.

Most chromosome disorders are not hereditary in the strict sense of the word but develop spontaneously and sporadically. Chromosomes of the parents usually are normal but an abnormality develops during the parents' production of male or female gametes (sperm or eggs) or during division of the fertilized egg. During cell division, an error may occur in the separation, recombination, or distribution of chromosomes to daughter cells.

Such is the case in the chromosome disorders Down syndrome (trisomy 21), trisomy 13, trisomy 18, fragile X syndrome, and cri du chat. Trisomies (presence of genetic material from three chromosomes of a similar type rather than the usual pair) 13 and 18 cause such major malformations, including those of the central nervous system, that these chromosome abnormalities are lethal.

Down syndrome
Down syndrome is the congenital form of retardation most familiar to the general population. It is the stereotype of mental retardation most commonly portrayed in print and film media.

In 1866, the English physician Langdon Down described a set of physical features associated with below-normal mental functioning. The children with such traits were referred to as having "mongolism" because of their slanted eyes, "epicanthal" folds of their eyelids, and flat nose. The term "mongoloid," now considered offensive and outdated, has been replaced by Down syndrome.

In 1959, a French physician Jerome Lejeune found an extra (i.e., 47th) chromosome in the cells of individuals with Down syndrome. Later determined to be a partial or complete chromosome 21, the disorder is now often referred to as "trisomy 21."

Down syndrome, the most common identifiable cause of mental retardation, occurs in 1 in 800–1,000 live births, although only two of ten fetuses with the syndrome are born alive. It accounts for at least 5–6% of all cases of mental retardation. Approximately 350,000 people with Down syndrome live in the United States, representing about 10% of all people in residential facilities.

Most people with Down syndrome exhibit moderate to severe retardation with only a few having an I.Q. above 50. Mental development usually proceeds relatively normally from birth to about six months of age. However, by age one year, I.Q. scores begin to drift gradually downward to about 30. The decline may be real, but the tests may not be sensitive enough to accurately predict intellectual functioning in infants and young children.

Studies indicate at least three chromosomal abnormalities can cause Down syndrome, nondisjunction, translocation, and mosaicism:

1. *Nondisjunction*, the most common cause of trisomy 21, occurs in 95% of cases. Individuals with this form of Down syndrome have 47 chromosomes instead of the normal 46.

They have an extra chromosome 21 because the pair of maternal chromosomes 21 failed to separate at the time of formation of the egg. Why nondisjunction occurs during gamete formation is unknown, but it occurs most often in older women. The risk of producing a child with the non-disjunction form of Down syndrome is approximately 1 in 100 births for women who are 32 years of age and increases to approximately 1 in 30 at 45 years of age. When actual numbers of pregnancies are considered, however, women under 35 years of age produce 80% of children with Down syndrome because they produce more children in general.

2. *Translocation* is the second most common cause of Down syndrome. The translocation occurs in the gamete either prior to or during conception when part of chromosome 21 breaks off during cell division and attaches to another chromosome—most commonly chromosome 15. This trans-location of a portion of chromosome 21 onto another chromosome results in cells with a total of 46 chromosomes but with extra genes from chromosome 21. The translocation form of Down syndrome occurs in only 1–2% of individuals with the disorder.

This form of Down syndrome is usually inherited from an unaffected "carrier" parent with only 45 chromosomes, but with an attached piece of chromosome 21 fused to chromosome 15. The attached portion of chromosome 21 provides the necessary genes for a full complement of genetic material so that the parent appears normal. Unaffected siblings of individuals with the translocation form of Down syndrome may have a chromosome pattern similar to the carrier parent.

3. The third and rarest cause of Down syndrome is due to somatic cell *mosaicism*, sometimes referred to as "incomplete" Down syndrome. It is responsible in only 1–2% of

cases. This form of the disorder is thought to be caused by uneven distribution of a chromosome 21 pair during a cell division that occurs in embryogenesis. In mosaicism, some of the child's cells will have one pair of chromosome 21 while other cells will show trisomy. Individuals with mosaic Down syndrome may exhibit a milder form of the disorder with less mental impairment and fewer medical complications.

What is the risk of having a second child with Down syndrome? It varies with the type of genetic abnormality that produced the syndrome. When nondisjunction or mosaicism is the culprit, the risk of producing a second child with Down syndrome is about 1 in 100. When the syndrome is caused by a translocation, however, the risk rises substantially to almost one in three. For this reason, genetic counseling is strongly advised for prospective parents who have already produced a child with Down syndrome.

The diagnosis of Down syndrome is not always made in newborn infants. The diagnosis is more easily made in older children. More than 100 physical signs are described in Down syndrome, but rarely are they all evident in one individual. The degree of mental retardation does not correlate with the number of physical signs of Down syndrome present.

The life expectancy of people with Down syndrome, once only about 12 years, has increased to about 40 years for those who receive modern medical care. Still, individuals with Down syndrome are at risk for many associated health problems: congenital heart disease (40%), gastrointestinal abnormalities (12%), nystagmus (i.e., abnormal side-to-side eye movement; 30%), congenital cataracts (3%), myopia (nearsightedness), conductive hearing loss (resulting from multiple ear infections), and hypothyroidism (congenital or developing later).

Table 1.4 Common Signs of Down Syndrome

Short stature

Small, flattened skull

Abundant neck skin

Flat, broad face with high cheek bones and small ears and nose

Short, broad hands with in-curving fingers

Upward slanting of the eyes with folds of skins (epicanthic folds) at the inside corner of the eye

Small mouth and short roof of mouth, which may cause the tongue to protrude and may contribute to articulation difficulties in speech

Single crease across the palm (so-called "simian" crease)

Reduced muscle tone (hypotonia) and hyperflexibility of joints

Heart defects (occur in about 1/3 of cases)

Increased susceptibility to upper respiratory infections

Incomplete or delayed sexual development

According to many clinicians, children with Down syndrome tend to be calm, cooperative, and adaptive. When they reach adolescence, however, they may experience emotional and behavioral difficulties. Occasionally, they present with psychotic disorders. Early diagnosis and early intervention techniques to bolster their physical and mental development can be of significant benefit.

People with Down syndrome often experience a decline in language, memory, problem-solving abilities, and self-care skills beginning in their thirties. Autopsies of individuals with Down syndrome over the age of 40 show a high incidence of senile plaques and neurofibrillary tangles in the brain. These are the same features associated with Alzheimer disease (the most common form of dementia in the general population) occurring at a later age in the general population. The association between the two disorders is not surprising, since both are related to abnormalities of chromosome 21.

Down syndrome can be diagnosed prior to birth by maternal screening or fetal diagnostic tests. Maternal screening tests generally measure quantities of various substances in the blood (alpha-fetoprotein, human chorionic gonadotropin, and unconjugated estriol). Results are compared with the mother's age to estimate the risk of producing a child with Down syndrome. Screening tests are usually offered between 15 and 20 weeks of gestation. Screening tests, unfortunately, detect only about 60% of fetuses with Down syndrome and false positive results occur frequently.

Fetal diagnostic tests examine the chromosomes of fetal cells, which are obtained by chorionic villus sampling (CVS), amniocentesis, or percutaneous umbilical blood sampling (PUBS). Each of these procedures carries a small risk of inducing miscarriage. Unlike the maternal tests, the fetal tests have a high degree of accuracy, about 98–99%. Amniocentesis is usually performed between 12 and 20 weeks of gestation, CVS between eight and 12 weeks, and PUBS after 20 weeks.

Fragile X syndrome

The second most common single cause of retardation (after Down syndrome) is fragile X syndrome, also known as Martin-Bell syndrome. This disorder is usually categorized as a chromosomal disorder because of what appears to be a pinched section on the long arm of the X chromosome. Research has identified a recessive mutation at a specific gene site on the X chromosome. The so-called "fragile site" (subject to breakage) occurs in about 1 in 1,500 males and about 1 in 1,000 females in the general population. The defective gene (FMR1) may be present in some cells and not in others (see chapter 9).

Much variability exists in the symptoms of fragile X syndrome, so misdiagnosis is common. Although the syndrome is generally associated with mental retardation, some individuals may be of normal intelligence. Retardation, when present, may range from mild to severe. The intellectual function of individuals with fragile X syndrome appears to decline during puberty.

The syndrome is fully expressed in boys more often than girls because girls (with their pair of X chromosomes) usually are protected by the low penetrance of the abnormal gene. As many as one third of females with the fragile X site may be partially affected with mild learning disabilities whether or not they exhibit the typical physical characteristics and associated mild mental retardation (see table 1.5).

Fragile X syndrome can be diagnosed before birth, although prenatal screening of maternal blood is reliable in only half of cases. Chromosomal, cytogenetic, or DNA testing of infant blood samples at some period after birth yields more reliable results. DNA testing reveals both the presence of the disorder and carriers of the disorder. All women of childbearing age who have a child diagnosed with fragile X syndrome are carriers for FMR1 gene expansion and are at increased risk of successive reproductive impairments. Any woman who

Table 1.5 Common Signs of Fragile X Syndrome

Short stature

Large head with long, thin face and long, soft ears

Prominent forehead

Long, soft hands

Hyperextensible joints ("double-jointed") in fingers

Postpubertal large testicles

knows that the syndrome is present in her family or who has unexplained mental retardation in her family should be tested and have genetic counseling prior to or soon after becoming pregnant.

Rett syndrome

Rett syndrome, described in 1966 by Andreas Rett, is a disorder found exclusively in females, occurring in 1 in 10,000–23,000 live female births. The syndrome occurs sporadically in 99.5% of cases, usually only once in a family, because affected individuals are so impaired they do not reproduce. In the rare instances when more than one child is affected, they are almost always identical twins or sisters.

Researchers had long reasoned that the responsible gene is located on the X chromosome, and its location was eventually narrowed down to the long arm of the X chromosome. Later researchers located the gene which they named MECP2. This gene produces an enzyme required for correct translation of the DNA template to daughter cells during cell division. An abnormal gene at the MECP2 site produces aberrations in the X chromosome that are usually lethal prior to birth in boys (who have no second X chromosome and thus no chance for a normal allele of the gene).

DNA testing is available to identify the Rett mutation in research laboratories, but the availability of the test is limited by time and resources. General clinical screening for the disorder is therefore not yet readily available.

In girls, a mosaic pattern with respect to expression of the abnormal MECP2 gene exists, and the severity of Rett syndrome is directly associated with the percentage of cells that express it. If random inactivation happens to the X chromosome carrying the mutated gene in a large proportion of cells, the symptoms will be mild. On the other hand, when a larger percentage of the cells have the healthy X chromosome turned off, the onset of Rett syndrome symptoms will be earlier and more severe.

Rett syndrome is classified as a pervasive developmental disorder (PDD), but a component of mental retardation often coexists. Rett syndrome is also associated with serious progressive neurological disability. Girls with this syndrome appear to develop normally until they are approximately five months of age. From that point until they are about four years old, their head growth slows down as compared with their normal peers. Deterioration in communication skills, motor skills, and social functioning starts at about one year of age. By the time they are 2 1/2 to 3 years old, a loss of purposeful hand movements occurs and a characteristic "hand-washing" mannerism begins.

Affected girls experience additional symptoms of neurological damage: ataxia (poor balance), tremor, uncoordinated gait, teeth-grinding, loss of speech, intermittent hyperventilation and a disorganized breathing pattern while awake, progressive scoliosis (crooked spine), and seizures.

Deterioration is rapid at the onset but slows later. By middle childhood, girls with Rett syndrome experience severe spasticity. Although some skills may eventually be regained, development of cerebral atrophy is common.

Prader-Willi syndrome

In Prader-Willi syndrome the chromosome abnormality is transmitted by the father, an example of the previously described gene imprinting or "parent of origin" effect. In 80% of cases (1 in 10,000 live births), the culprit is a deletion of paternal copies of one, two, or more contiguous genes on chromosome 15. Over 90% of cases are sporadic. This is one of the five most common syndromes seen in birth defects clinics.

Prader-Willi syndrome was probably first described by Langdon Down in 1887, but the syndrome is named for two of the three men who identified the set of symptoms in 1956. Prader-Willi syndrome results in I.Q. varying between 20 and 85 (i.e., from severe mental retardation to low normal intelligence) and compulsive, indiscriminate eating behavior. The preoccupation with eating is so compelling that the comment has been made that, for a Prader-Willi child, "life is one endless meal." Compulsive eating often leads to obesity and to the complications associated with severe obesity on a small, fragile skeletal frame (e.g., fractures). Individuals with Prader-Willi syndrome commonly require constant supervision in order to limit them to a reasonable caloric intake. Otherwise, they may steal food and even eat food that is unpalatable to others. Many will get up at night to seek food. They are frequently cunning in their attempts to obtain food and become easily frustrated and angry when deterred.

In addition to eating behavior, individuals with Prader-Willi syndrome often exhibit oppositional and defiant behavior with emotional ability, irritability, and tantrums. They frequently engage in obsessional thinking and compulsive behaviors that often include masturbation and self-injury. Skin-picking is the most common form of self-injury in people with Prader-Willi syndrome; however, they may also engage in nose picking, nail biting, lip biting, rectal digging, and hair pulling.

Other compulsive behaviors may include checking-rechecking, hand washing, counting, symmetrical arrangement, and insistence on sameness in the environment. Interpersonal problems are common, especially in older children and adults with Prader-Willi syndrome. They differ from other groups of individuals with mental retardation in exhibiting less sexual acting out behavior.

Table 1.6 Common Signs of Prader-Willi Syndrome

Small stature
Small skeletal frame
Hypotonia
Soft, poor teeth
Thick saliva
Small hands and feet
Hypogonadism (underdeveloped sex organs)
Soft, easily broken bones

Angelman syndrome

Angelman syndrome was initially described in 1965 by Harry Angelman. The rare syndrome is associated with mental retardation (with I.Q. at 50 or less) and characteristic physical appearance and behavior. Like Prader-Willi syndrome, Angelman syndrome demonstrates the parent of origin inheritance pattern. Angelman syndrome is caused by the same small deletion on chromosome 15 as exists in Prader-Willi syndrome, except that the defect is inherited from the mother. Despite the fact that both syndromes are caused by a similar mutation on chromosome 15, they have different presentations because maternal and paternal copies of the gene play different roles in development.

The frequency of Angelman syndrome is unknown but the condition is thought to be rare. The families of these individuals seem to be at high risk for producing another child with Angelman syndrome, which is to be expected since the parent is a carrier.

The overall level of mental retardation associated with Angelman syndrome is in the severe to profound range. Psychological testing, especially intelligence testing, may be difficult to administer and to interpret because of difficulties in speech and coordination. Comprehension is significantly better than expressive speech in these individuals.

In general, children with Angelman syndrome (sometimes referred to as the "happy puppet" syndrome because of the associated jerky gait) appear to be happy and sociable with frequent, spontaneous, and often inappropriate laughter. Hand flapping may occur during periods of excitement. Frequent nighttime awakening is characteristic (see table 1.7).

Cri du chat syndrome

Cri du chat (cat cry) syndrome is caused by deletion (varying in size) of part of the short arm of chromosome 5. Children with cri du chat syndrome exhibit severe mental retardation (with I.Q. less than 50) and a cat-like cry in infancy that disappears with age. The characteristic sound is caused by an abnormal larynx.

Table 1.7 Common Signs of Angelman Syndrome

Small head with wide and smiling mouth, a thin upper lip, pointed chin, and prominent tongue
Fair hair and skin (approximately 1/2 of cases)
Blue eyes (most of cases)
Strabismus ("crossed eyes," approximately 2/3 of cases)

Table 1.8 Common Signs of Cri du Chat Syndrome

Small head with low set ears
Slanted eyes
Wide brow with abnormally wide space between eyes and eyebrows
Abnormally small jaws

Children with cri du chat syndrome exhibit growth retardation, mental retardation, and often show signs of multiple chromosomal abnormalities. Most do not live into adulthood; thus, most cases are caused by de novo deletions. Approximately 12% result from unbalanced translocations or recombinations of a chromosome 5 transmitted by one of the parents.

Cornelia de Lange Syndrome

Cornelia de Lange syndrome is a disorder of unknown biochemical and genetic basis, recognized by characteristic physical abnormalities (especially facial) and the presence of mental retardation (OMIM). The syndrome was originally described in 1933 by the Dutch pediatrician for whom the syndrome is named. At one time, the name "Amsterdam dwarf" was used, but the name was discontinued because short stature is not invariably a feature of the syndrome.

Cornelia de Lange syndrome occurs in approximately 1 in 40,000–100,000 live births and affects boys and girls equally. Its exact mode of transmission is unknown. Several chromosomal abnormalities have been suggested, but a site on chromosome 3 has been the area most frequently implicated. Most cases occur sporadically, although familial inheritance patterns have occasionally been reported. Both autosomal dominant and autosomal recessive inheritance patterns have been suggested based on studies of different affected families, although the dominant pattern may be more common.

Infants with Cornelia de Lange syndrome demonstrate failure to thrive as well as problems with regurgitation, vomiting, and swallowing so that aspiration pneumonia is a frequent problem early in life. Physically, they exhibit growth failure and abnormalities of face, hair, and extremities. Sixty percent of individuals with Cornelia de Lange syndrome will experience significant hearing loss and thus develop speech delays.

Table 1.9 Common Signs of Cornelia de Lange Syndrome

Small stature (common but not invariable)

Distinctive facial features, with eyebrows that are characteristically well-defined, arched, and fan out laterally to join in the middle of the forehead above the bridge of the nose

Long and curled eyelashes (frequent)

Small and upturned nose, with a long philtrum

Mouth is turned down with thin lips

Limb abnormalities ranging from small limbs to severe reduction in the size of limbs, primarily the arms

Single transverse palmar crease on the hand and malformations of the fingers; webbing of second and third toes

Heavy body hair

Hearing loss

Multiple other physical abnormalities such as bowel duplication or malformation and congenital heart disease

The majority of individuals with Cornelia de Lange syndrome who live beyond 13 years of age will experience onset of puberty; often females will have normal menstrual cycles.

Individuals usually exhibit severe mental retardation, but occasionally will demonstrate borderline or normal intelligence. I.Q. estimates range from below 30 up to 86 with an average of 53. Those with higher I.Q. tend to have more normal weight and head circumference at birth. Severe limitations in speech capability are typical, ranging from absence of speech to use of single words and may be due, in part, to hearing problems.

Behaviorally, children with Cornelia de Lange syndrome avoid being held and exhibit stereotypical movements, including twirling behavior. Their temperaments vary. Some are described as "placid and good natured" while others are irritable, destructive, and self-abusive (frequently in the form of finger biting). Bruxism (i.e., teeth grinding) is common.

Because most cases of Cornelia de Lange syndrome are sporadic, the exact risk of producing a child with the disorder is unknown but appears to be negligible when both parents are normal. If one parent is mildly affected, the risk rises to 50%. However, most adults with Cornelia de Lange syndrome do not have children due to the severity of their disability.

Multifactorial Disorders

Multifactorial disorders are those determined by the interaction of several genes with each other and with nongenetic factors such as nutrition, infection, and toxic agents. These disorders are very common and are involved in the majority of birth defects, where the intrauterine environment may play a role. Such defects include spina bifida and anencephaly (absence of significant brain development), cleft lip and palate, clubfoot, and congenital heart defects. Some combinations of abnormal genes and environmental factors can lead to mental retardation.

In utero influences
The environment in the uterus has a profound impact, both physically and intellectually, on the development of the child. Detrimental prenatal influences include insufficient blood flow to the fetus causing inadequate oxygen and nutrients and inadequate removal of waste products; presence of toxic chemicals ingested or inhaled by the mother (i.e., alcohol, medications, drugs, lead, pollutants from the water and food supply, etc.); injuries to the mother (such as trauma causing blood loss or uterine damage) causing simultaneous injuries to the fetus; compromised health of the mother (poor general health, severe hypothyroidism, poorly controlled diabetes mellitus, AIDS,

syphilis, and toxoplasmosis); and Rh-factor blood incompatibility between mother and fetus.

Viral infections in pregnant women can cause abnormalities in the developing fetus. The earlier in the pregnancy the infection occurs, the more likely and more severe is the effect on the fetus. The classic example is congenital rubella. Rubella ("German measles") is a relatively mild viral infection in children and adults; however, it can cause severe difficulties in fetuses. When a woman contracts rubella during the first month of pregnancy, her fetus has a 50% risk for significant birth defects, including mental retardation. Infection in the third month of pregnancy carries a 15% risk for birth defects.

Birth defects (spina bifida, anencephaly, etc.) may be more common in twin or multiple births for various reasons, including compromised placental blood flow to one (or more) of the fetuses.

Nutritional factors

Nutritional deficiencies can be of concern in both the prenatal and the postnatal period. A malnourished pregnant woman will deliver a malnourished infant. The first two trimesters of pregnancy (i.e., the first six months of gestation) are the most critical in the development of the infant's nervous system, including the brain. Malnutrition of the mother during this critical period can result in mental impairment in the child. Vitamin deficiencies, especially deficiency of the B vitamin folate, can produce neurological damage to the fetus—including spina bifida (incomplete closure of the spine during prenatal development), anencephaly (failure of brain development), and mental retardation.

Folic acid must be taken within the first four weeks of pregnancy to be an effective preventive. Unfortunately, women may not realize that they are pregnant until the second month of gestation and after neurological damage to the fetus may have occurred. For this reason, women must consider regular dietary supplements during childbearing years. A 1998 report of the Institute of Medicine recommended daily supplements of 400 micrograms of folic acid for sexually active women of reproductive age.

Delivery and postnatal factors

Events occurring just before, during, or just after delivery of a child can significantly impact its physical and intellectual well-being. Prematurity and low birth weight are two such perinatal conditions. Although many children who come into the world early and many who have low birth weights develop normally both physically and intellectually, significant developmental problems can occur in some, including low intellectual functioning.

During childbirth, the most important factor that can cause neurological damage (and potentially mental retardation) in the child is inadequate oxygen (hypoxia) or absolute lack of oxygen (anoxia). These can result from situations such as prolonged or very short labor or delivery causing compression of the umbilical cord or brain trauma, misplacement or knotting of the umbilical cord around the neck or under the arm, or breech birth presentation. Premature birth can also cause hypoxia in infants with poorly developed lungs. The delivery itself can cause traumatic injury to the infant's brain (and possibly result in mental retardation), especially when forceps must be used to guide the head through the birth canal.

During the newborn period (the time from birth until the infant is around four weeks old), the most important infection from the point of view of disturbing normal development is herpes simplex type 2. Herpes simplex type 2 is a sexually transmitted disease (STD) that can be controlled, but not cured, in adults. Women with this STD run the risk of infecting their newborn during vaginal delivery so that the neonate may develop herpes simplex encephalitis (infection of brain tissue) within two weeks of birth. This form of encephalitis can cause devastating brain damage and mental retardation. Early treatment of infected neonates with an antiviral medication may prevent the serious effects.

Events that occur during childhood also can lead to disability. Some authorities estimate that in as many as 15% of children with mild mental retardation the causative factor is trauma or neglect. Head trauma accounts for most of these. It is estimated that as many as 1 in 30 newborns sustains significant head trauma before reaching adulthood.

In children, adolescents, and teenagers the majority of head injuries result from falls, bicycle accidents, motor vehicle accidents, and sports-related injuries—although child abuse victims may suffer brain injury from being shaken violently. Boys are twice as likely as girls to sustain significant head trauma and thus more likely to develop the trauma-induced form of mental retardation. The age of highest risk for such injuries is between 15 and 25 years. The most common cause of serious head injuries in this group is motor vehicle accidents. Those individuals below the age of 18 years who suffer head injury resulting in significantly diminished intellectual capacity are, by definition, mentally retarded.

Lead poisoning can lead to neurological problems and mental retardation. Lead ingestion may occur when a child ingests chips from old house paint. Lead can also enter the system through inhalation when older buildings are renovated. (Federal regulations now require that commercial paints contain no lead.) Other causes of lead poisoning may include heavy exposure to old batteries, repeated inhalation of leaded gasoline, and prolonged ingestion of water carried in old lead pipes.

The most important substance of abuse that can cause birth defects is ethanol (drinking alcohol). Excessive alcohol intake during pregnancy is the cause of fetal alcohol syndrome (FAS). The American Academy of Pediatrics (AAP) reports that, in industrialized countries, FAS occurs in approximately 2.5% of newborns. According to pediatrician Alan Greene, FAS is responsible for 10–20% of cases of mental retardation with I.Q. in the 50–80 range (average, 63).

FAS is probably the most common identifiable cause of mental retardation that is preventable. When pregnant women drink alcohol, even in small amounts, their unborn children are at high risk for developing abnormalities of three main types: distortion of facial features, growth retardation (including small head), and mental retardation. Milder forms of the condition, sometimes referred to as "fetal alcohol effects," can occur with abnormalities in only two of the three main areas. Poor academic performance and behavior problems are common in these children.

Prevention of this potentially disabling condition requires only that pregnant women, women who are considering pregnancy, and women of childbearing age who are sexually active refrain from consuming alcohol—a preventive measure that is simple, yet unlikely to be universally enacted given human nature.

What are the risks of using drugs during pregnancy?

Statistics suggest that the use of drugs, both prescription and "recreational" types, by pregnant women is increasing. Today, one of every ten newborns in the United States has experienced prenatal exposure to one or more drugs. The impact of prenatal illicit drug exposure on a newborn includes failure to thrive, low birth weight, irritability, growth retardation, and physical and intellectual deficits.

2. Normal Development

The template for normal human development allows for variation within limits. Students of human development have studied the process primarily by observation, laying down so-called "milestones of development" (Appendix B) as guides to predicting the acquisition of intellectual and motor abilities over time. Human development does not cease with puberty, but continues throughout life so long as the brain and body are reasonably healthy. The theories of normal human development provide the background for understanding abnormalities, including mental retardation, and the impact of those abnormalities on the lives of those affected.

Jean Piaget and Human Development

Jean Piaget, a Swiss psychologist credited by many as being the foremost figure in twentieth century developmental psychology, was the first to make a systematic study of cognitive development (i.e., the acquisition of learning and understanding) in children. A student of Carl Jung, Piaget became interested in how children learn. He developed his theories based on his observations of his own children.

Piaget believed the minds of children evolve through a series of stages, constantly creating and recreating their own sense of reality at each stage of their lives. This process entails integrating simple concepts with progressively more complex concepts. According to Piaget, the sequence of stages is not automatic but depends on evolution of the central nervous system and on life experiences.

Piaget believed that nature provides a biological template for the development of children's ability to think, to learn, and to reason. The template he described was divided into four stages of cognitive development each of which must be successfully negotiated before progressing to the next stage: sensorimotor, preoperational, concrete operational, and formal operational.

Sensorimotor stage (birth to two years old)

The first two years of life are devoted chiefly to preoccupation with the five senses, mastering physical reflexes, and learning basic motor control to seek pleasurable or interesting experiences. Infants learn early to recognize sounds and smells and shortly thereafter to recognize faces, especially those associated with pleasure or with pain. During this first stage, they also become aware of themselves as a separate entity and realize that the objects around them are separate but consistently present.

This sensorimotor stage of development is made possible by the brain's "prewiring" that allows recognition of different stimuli and their connections with multiple perceptions.

Preoperational stage (ages two to six or seven years)

In the second stage, children develop symbolic thinking; that is, they learn to represent objects by words and to use words to convey wishes, fears, or activity. At this stage, children's thought patterns are dominated by magical thinking and a belief that experiences may be directly related to objects, time, or events only coincidentally present at the time of the experience. Attention span and memory are limited. Pretend play and fanciful thinking are common, as are imaginary friends and talking animals and toys.

The preoperational stage appears to be dependent upon the genetically determined capacity for language, but environmental factors—such as parental responses to attempts at communication—are clearly important in enhancing this capacity and teaching children to acquire new words, combine words with appropriate meaning and syntax, and develop correct language structure.

Concrete operational stage (ages seven to eleven or twelve years)
Children begin to form patterns of logical thinking from mid-childhood until puberty. They also begin to classify objects by similarities and differences, to develop a sense of time, and to understand numerical concepts. They begin to shift from a concept of themselves as the center of the universe to the realization that other people and their differing perspectives have validity. Children acquire a more logical form of reasoning and develop better understanding of cause and effect, including complex causal sequences of events, abilities required for successful transition into an academic environment and later into adulthood.

Formal operational stage (ages twelve years into adulthood)
Piaget's fourth stage is characterized by orderliness of thinking and mastery of logical thought processes. These allow for a more flexible approach to mental experimentation. As their fund of knowledge increases exponentially, adolescents learn to manipulate abstract concepts, to develop hypotheses, and to realize the implications of their own thinking and the thoughts of others. New levels of problem-solving ability are achieved.

L. A. Breger and Human Development

In 1974, L. A. Breger proposed that human development incorporates three key precepts:

1. Behavioral maturation proceeds from the simple to the complex,

2. Future behaviors, whether temporally near or distant, are a product of their antecedents (i.e., prior responses to the environment), and

3. The human response to a particular event or experience often depends on the developmental stage at which the experience occurs.

Biological Aspects of Brain Development

The human brain contains 1,000,000,000,000 (one trillion) nerve cells and a thousand trillion intercellular connections. The brain's independent nerve cells and their interconnections cooperate in the abstract process we know as "thought" while simultaneously operating an indispensable relay system that coordinates basic functions of the body. This complex system works in a superbly efficient manner most of the time, a state we label "normal."

Brain growth is essential in normal human development. At birth, the brain is almost one third of adult size. It grows rapidly during the first years of life, reaching 60% of adult size by the first year and 90% of adult size by the end of the fifth year. The remaining 10% of the brain's growth occurs in the next ten years so that the brain reaches its full weight by the time the individual is 16 years old.

First 20 weeks of gestation
We divide the development of the human brain before birth into two stages. The first stage occurs in the first 20 weeks of gestational life during which time the organs and nervous system begin to develop. Nests of primordial cells produce immature nerve cells that migrate to preordained

portions of the developing brain. By the end of the first four months of gestation the human brain has established its basic architecture, with cells of the most primitive parts of the brain (the brain stem) organizing first while those of the most advanced portions of the brain (the cerebral cortex) follow shortly afterward. Most of the nerve cells in the cerebral cortex are produced by 20 weeks of gestation.

Non-neuronal cells called "glial cells" also develop in the early days of prenatal life. Glial cells help guide the immature neurons in their migration to their assigned destinations.

Second 20 weeks of gestation

The second stage of human brain development occurs in the last 20 weeks of gestation when the brain continues to enlarge, primarily due to the proliferation of glial cells. Multiple connections (axons and dendrites) between nerve cells develop. A thin, protective coating called a myelin sheath is formed by glial cells and envelops the developing axons, insulating them and improving their capacity to carry the electrical discharges that trigger the myriads of chemical processes by which neurons function.

While the brain grows rapidly during prenatal life and for the first year after birth, different portions of the brain and central nervous system grow at different rates. Those portions of the brain growing most rapidly are the most vulnerable to damage. Insults to rapidly growing regions of the brain before birth can result in mental retardation and cerebral palsy.

By the time of birth, the growth of the spinal cord, the brain stem, and much of the forebrain (portions of the brain that sit on top of the brain stem) is largely complete. The cerebral cortex and the cerebellar cortex, on the other hand, continue development into the first year of life. The myelin sheath that covers nerve axons and increases the speed at which they can conduct impulses continues development in school-age children and probably continues until early adult life.

Cerebral Cortex

The cerebral cortex is the most advanced portion of the brain and the key portion that makes us human. It is the area involved in the brain's most complex functions, including language and thought. The cerebral cortex in humans has a total surface area ten times that of the cerebral cortex of rhesus monkeys.

The cerebral cortex makes up only about 3 percent of the brain in the earliest days of gestation. By the time of birth, however, it forms 67 percent of the entire brain. The cerebral cortex is about two millimeters thick. Within that two millimeters are six distinct layers containing different types of neurons and neurotransmitters with differing connections to various parts of the brain.

The cerebral cortex is divided front to back into two halves (hemispheres), with each possessing four relatively symmetrical anatomical regions that have specialized functions. The regions are interconnected so that one region may be able to partially compensate for another that is damaged, although those regions on the left side of the brain tend to be dominant in controlling higher brain activities. These distinct regions, located on each half of the brain, are known as lobes: frontal, parietal, temporal, and occipital.

The frontal lobes form the area of the brain behind the forehead and the eyes. They are the largest of the lobes and contain almost one third of the brain's surface. The frontal lobes determine how people act on information. They are the seat of what is called the brain's "executive functions." These functions include modulating emotion as well as conceptualizing, planning, prioritizing, implementing, sequencing, and monitoring complex behaviors.

The frontal lobes are where abstract thoughts are formed and such concepts as awareness, identity, and morality reside. The frontal lobes also contain the major areas of the brain that deal with voluntary body movements and speech. In most people, even most left-handers, the left hemisphere is dominant; thus, most primary speech functions are controlled by the left frontal lobe. Some researchers believe that the capacity for working memory (both immediate recall and recent memory) is localized predominantly in the left frontal cortex, although bilateral frontal cortex lesions usually are required for working memory to be severely impaired.

Frontal lobe dysfunction usually results in impairment in motivation, attention span, and sequencing of actions and can cause slowed thinking, poor judgment, apathy, decreased curiosity, social withdrawal, irritability, and sudden explosions of impulsive disinhibition. Frontal lobe dysfunction can be difficult to detect on standard neuropsychological tests because the I.Q. of an affected individual may be only marginally affected (activities that are measured for estimations of I.Q. are primarily functions of the parietal lobes). Frontal lobe dysfunction may become readily apparent only in unstructured, stressful situations.

The parietal lobes are located behind the frontal lobes and under the top of the skull. They are primarily involved with interpreting and integrating information obtained through the five senses—smell, taste, vision, hearing, and touch—as well as imparting awareness of the body's location in its immediate space. As noted above, the ability of the brain to coordinate, categorize, and utilize multiple pieces of data appears to be a function of the so-called "association" areas of the parietal lobe. These are the abilities that are measured on standard I.Q. tests.

The temporal lie adjacent to the temples and the ears and stretch toward the back of the brain. They are involved with emotional reactivity and processing of sounds and smells. The temporal lobes are critical to the formation of memories.

The occipital lobes, located at the back of the brain beneath the back of the skull, are the smallest of the lobes and are primarily concerned with vision.

Sub-cortical regions of the brain, located below the cerebral cortex, are more primitive than the cerebral cortex, but their functions are intricately interwoven with those of the cerebral cortex so that damage to them prior to birth often results in developmental disorders in children.

The hypothalamus is the deep brain structure that serves as the major way station for many of the brain's activities. It is interconnected with almost all parts of the brain. The hypothalamus controls essential bodily functions such as temperature, eating, drinking, and reproduction, as well as regulation of the endocrine glands.

The limbic system, often labeled the "seat of human emotion," is a complex, interconnected circuit of brain structures involved in emotional responses. The circuit includes the hypothalamus and its prominent connections to the frontal and temporal lobes of the brain. The circuit is intricately involved with complex emotions such as pleasure, friendliness, love, and affection as well as more primitive emotions such as fear, anger, rage, aversion, and aggression.

The basal ganglia are nerve centers buried deep within the brain. Their interconnection with the cerebral cortex has major implications for behavior. They are particularly involved in voluntary movement. Damage to the basal ganglia often results in movement disorders and may result in compulsive forms of behavior.

The amygdala, a pair of nerve centers located deep within the cerebral hemispheres, form part of the limbic system. The amygdala receive fibers from all sensory areas and appear to act as an important gate for integrating internal stimuli (such as hunger and thirst) and external stimuli (such as pain and pleasure) and attaching emotional significance to memories. Thus, the amygdala appear to rate the importance of an emotional experience and activate other portions of the limbic system accordingly. This allows an emotionally intense stimulus to be firmly etched into the memory while less intense stimuli may be quickly discarded.

The amygdala also appear to be the mediators of learned fear responses, such as anxiety and panic, and may translate these emotions by producing corresponding affects (facial and postural expressions). The amygdala have a more powerful influence on the cerebral cortex (stimulating or suppressing cortical activity) than the cortex has on the amygdala.

Destruction of the amygdala appears to eliminate the ability of individuals to distinguish fear and anger in other people's voices and facial expressions while preserving their ability to recognize happiness, sadness, or disgust.

The cerebellum is a separate portion of the brain attached to the brain stem and located beneath the back portion of the cerebral cortex. The cerebellum functions primarily in coordinating gross motor movements. Damage to the cerebellum may cause spasticity of movement.

Neurological Development

Different portions of the human brain mature at different times well into the second decade. As a result, different brain functions mature at different rates. In addition, people mature at different rates so that a "range of normal" is usually defined for the acquisition of major developmental skills.

In general, the development of major skills proceeds in two directions: from head to foot and from the center of the body outward toward the tips of the extremities. The first muscles that babies learn to control are those of the mouth and the eyes.

Next, babies learn to hold their head erect and to use their arms. Their first attempts at moving their arms amount to gross flailing motions, but they gradually gain mastery over those limbs and by nine or ten months can pick up pea-sized objects using thumbs and index fingers. By the age of nine months babies can sit alone; by twelve months, they can take steps with one hand held. By 15 months they can walk independently, and by the middle of their second year they are almost outrunning their parents.

Language Development

Language development begins with single one- and two-syllable words, such as "mama" or "dada," which initially have little meaning to infants until they realize that those verbalizations cause the faces of nurturing presences to light up dramatically. The entities attached to those happy faces, in turn, react by producing pleasant sensations for baby's enjoyment.

By the end of the first year, babies can say a handful of meaningful single words. Over the next six months, they acquire new words at the rate of about one word per month until a burst of linguistic activity occurs in the middle of the second year and the vocabulary increases rapidly. By the end of the second year, toddlers can speak combinations of words and begin making three-word sentences. Some otherwise normal toddlers (more commonly boys) do not demonstrate this capacity until the end of the third year but then go on to acquire normal language skills.

As children enter their third year, they begin using sentences with more complex structure. The various parts of speech are acquired in approximately the following order: nouns, verbs, adjectives, adverbs, pronouns, and prepositions. Three-year-old children are usually well into the pronoun and preposition stage.

Articulation of words develops slowly at first. Some baby talk in young children (and their adoring parents) is expected during the first two to three years. By age two years, children produce about one third of sounds correctly. This progressively improves so that, by age six, children can pronounce 90% of sounds correctly.

Children should be producing grammatically correct sentences by the time they are four or five years old. They should be able to relate simple messages by the time they are four, and their speech should be understandable to people outside their family by the time they are five years old.

Stuttering is common among young children when they first begin to put words together into phrases. Stuttering usually appears intermittently until it finally disappears around the fifth year of life. When stuttering is brief and transient, it is considered to be a phase of normal development.

Temperament and Social Reactivity

Babies come into the world with differing degrees of reactivity and irritability. A stable pattern of temperament usually is not established until the second year of life.

Healthy babies are socially interactive from the first days of life. They form a strong bond with their primary caretakers within the first few weeks. Between seven and nine months of age, infants begin to protest separation from their parents and react negatively to the approach of strangers.

Sex differences in behavior begin to emerge by two years of age. Although some of the differences may result from cultural influence, the consistency of sex differences in preferred activities argues for the presence of biological causes. Boys tend to be more aggressive and to play with toys that can be manipulated. Girls tend to prefer doll play and artwork. By the end of the third year, children prefer to play with other children of the same sex.

Young children initially prefer parallel play; that is, they play alongside other children but do not interact in play with them. Cooperative play emerges later and with it comes a tendency to play "make believe." During school years the role of peers become predominant in shaping social behavior. Children play in small groups and form "clubs." They enjoy shared activities such as collecting things. They also like to share secrets and make up rules to share within their small groups. Social humor develops; personal appearance and dress become important symbols of belonging. With the onset of adolescence, peer pressure becomes of paramount importance as teenagers wrestle with academic, social, and cultural demands while tackling a completely new tangle of issues involving sexuality.

Moral Development

Moral development also progresses from childhood through adulthood. Infants live in a world that is free of moral directives. They are, in effect, happy little hedonists. By the second year of life, however, children begin to experience embarrassment, shame, and guilt, demonstrating the emergence of a rudimentary code of moral behavior. By the third year, children begin to internalize parental standards even when their parents are not available to provide cues. The importance of rules and adhering to them becomes apparent in elementary-school-age children. The moral codes of these children tend to be absolute with no gray zones between right and wrong, with strong consequences for anyone who breaks the rules. Boys are generally more rigid than girls in this respect.

The elaboration of more complex moral principles is a gradual and not necessarily sequential process that occurs during the teenage years. The process ultimately leads to the conviction that moral principles of justice should supercede man-made laws.

Developmental Milestones

While parents watch the development of their young children closely, convinced that theirs are the best and brightest of children, judgments regarding intellectual potential based on early developmental milestones should be made with extreme caution. Children who develop mental retardation, either from genetic causes or through insults to their developing brain, often exhibit delayed or incomplete acquisition of intellectual, language, social, and motor skills as compared with normal children. The younger children are, however, the less value standard developmental milestones have in predicting intelligence. In particular, gross motor milestones can be very misleading and are not intended as absolute predictors of future performance. Language development is generally a more accurate predictor of intellectual capability in children. (See Appendix B.)

3. Evolving Concepts of Mental Retardation

Mental retardation is by no means new. It neither emerged in response to the increasing sophistication and demands of our modern educational system nor suddenly erupted due to environmental pollution so prevalent in 20th century civilization. Mental retardation has always been with us.

Mental Retardation and History

Historical references to mental retardation can be found as far back as the therapeutic papyri of Thebes (Luxor), Egypt, around 1552 B.C.E. The plight of mentally retarded people has been and still is dependent on the customs and beliefs of the culture. In ancient Greece in the city-state Sparta, neonates were examined by a state council of elders. If the child was found to be "defective," it was eliminated. In the second century C.E. in the Roman Empire, individuals with disabilities, including children, were frequently sold to be used for entertainment or amusement.

During the Middle Ages (5th to 15th centuries), more humane practices evolved (i.e., decrease in infanticide and the establishment of "foundling homes"), although the status and care of people with retardation varied greatly. Many were sold into slavery or abandoned. As early as the beginning of the 12th century, Henry II of England supported legislation that designated individuals with mental retardation as wards of the state, thereby extending some protection to them. Toward the end of that era, in 1690, John Locke published his famous work entitled *An Essay Concerning Human Understanding* proposing that individuals are born without innate ideas and that the mind is a "tabula rasa," a blank slate. This concept profoundly influenced the care and training provided to those with mental retardation. Locke was the first to distinguish between mental retardation and mental illness.

The work of physician Jean-Marc-Gaspard Itard was a cornerstone event in the evolution of treatment of mental retardation. In 1800, Itard was hired to work with the so-called "wild boy of Aveyron," a child who had lived his early life under primitive conditions and with a pack of canines in the woods of south central France. At the age of 12 years, the boy was sent to the Institute for Deaf-Mutes because Victor, as the boy was ultimately named, was a "savage" with limited hearing and no acquired speech.

Using the work of Locke and of Condillac (who emphasized the importance of learning through the senses), Itard developed a broad educational program for Victor focused on developing the boy's senses, intellect, and emotions and attempted to teach the boy basic living skills, including language. Although Victor apparently suffered from mental retardation, Itard was able to teach him the rudiments of social behavior. After five years of training, Victor continued to have significant difficulties in language and social interaction, but acquired more skills and knowledge than many of Itard's contemporaries believed possible. Itard's efforts stimulated new determination in Europe to educate people with mental retardation.

Supervised initially by Itard, Edouard Seguin devoted himself to working with children with mental retardation at the Hospice for Incurables in France. By the mid-19th century, he developed a comprehensive approach to their education known as the "Physiological Method." Assuming a direct relationship between the senses and cognition, Seguin's approach began with sensory training including vision, hearing, taste, smell, and eye-hand coordination. The curriculum extended from developing basic self-care skills to vocational education with an emphasis on perception, coordination, imitation, positive reinforcement, memory, and generalization.

In 1850 Seguin moved to the United States, where he became a driving force in the education of individuals with mental retardation. In 1876, he founded the Association of Medical Officers of American Institutions for Idiotic and Feeble Minded Persons, now known as the American Association on Mental Retardation (AAMR). Modifications of many of Seguin's techniques are still in use today.

Also in 1850, Wilhelm Griesinger, a prominent psychiatrist, published "Observations on Cretinism" and proposed that mental retardation has various causes. At the time, most people regarded mental retardation as a single condition.

In 1877, John L. H. Down made a seminal observation in his classic monograph, "The Mongolian Type of Idiocy." In that work, he described a subtype of mental retardation with distinctive physical features (later to be called Down syndrome). He went on to conclude that causes of mental retardation can be divided into three groups: congenital, developmental, and accidental.

After the publication of Down's work, many clinicians began a concerted search to identify specific conditions that could manifest as mental retardation. Although disorders such as tuberous sclerosis were subsequently identified, this advance in knowledge provided little benefit to those affected by mental retardation because no corresponding treatment advances accompanied the diagnostic advances. As a result, progress in the field of mental retardation was left to educators.

During the late nineteenth and the early twentieth centuries, mental retardation residential training schools proliferated. The increase in availability of this service was influenced by the availability of tests (primarily the intelligence or I.Q. test) to diagnose mental retardation and the belief that, with proper training, individuals with mental retardation could be "cured." By 1892, residential training schools were established in most states (19 state-operated and 9 privately operated centers).

In 1905, two French physicians, Alfred Binet and Theodore Simon, developed objective tests for estimating intelligence in children to determine which children needed specialized education. The newly developed test of intelligence was translated in 1908 by Henry Goddard, director of research at the training school in Vineland, New Jersey, who published an American version in 1910. Mass testing of individuals of all ages then began. Testing included individuals in the general population as well as those on the fringes of society and those who were incarcerated. Individuals in the latter groups tended to score in the mild range of mental retardation on Binet's test.

The unfortunate result was that mild mental retardation and "psychopathy" or criminal behavior began to be linked in the opinions of many policy makers. Widely read books, such as Goddard's "The Kallikaks," suggested that mental retardation and antisocial behavior were hereditary. Overemphasis on this point led some to view people with mild mental retardation as dangers to society through presumed "loose sexual behavior" and their production of equally impaired progeny. The eugenics movement (a philosophy advocating improving the genetic composition of the human race) sought to protect society from these evils by institutionalizing and sterilizing individuals with mental retardation, a practice that continued well into middle of the twentieth century.

Renewed interest in primary prevention of mental retardation began in 1934 with the identification by Ivar Folling of a form of mental retardation caused by the metabolic condition phenylketonuria (see page 13). Later researchers found that a modified diet given to infants and young children with this metabolic defect can prevent or reduce mental retardation. Thereafter, medical science again became interested in identifying biological causes of mental retardation and finding effective treatments for them. In 1961 Robert Guthrie developed a screening test for PKU.

In 1935 Edgar Doll developed the Vineland Social Maturity Scale to assess daily living skills and adaptive behavior of individuals suspected of having mental retardation.

During World War II, Nazis exterminated people with mental retardation as well as others who did not fit the Nazi "master race" image.

Following the war, clinicians believed strongly that primary preventive measures could be used effectively to reduce or eliminate physical and mental health problems and mental retardation. Institutions remained the primary focus of care for those individuals with mental retardation who were unable to remain within their family group, while special education programs for children with mental retardation in public schools increasingly became available.

In the 1950s, family groups began to organize as advocates for research in the field of mental retardation. In the United States, the National Association for Retarded Children (NARC) was formed. They provided strong influence on the panel of national experts appointed by President John F. Kennedy to study methods of prevention and treatment of mental illness and mental retardation so that, in 1963, the President called on Congress to establish a national program to combat mental retardation. The program brought together for the first time in the United States the biological, psychological, and educational specialists needed to focus on the study of mental retardation and its prevention and treatment.

By the 1960s it had become obvious that residential training schools were overcrowded and unable to "cure" mental retardation. As a result, many residents were moved back into society where the educational focus changed toward special education classes in local schools. The training schools then devolved into custodial living centers.

In the 1970s *Wyatt v. Stickney*, a landmark federal class action suit, established the right to treatment of individuals living in mental retardation residential facilities in Alabama. Purely custodial care was no longer acceptable anywhere in the United States. Following the decision the United States Congress passed the 1975 Education for the Handicapped Act. Now titled the Individuals with Disabilities Education Act (IDEA), the legislation guarantees the appropriate education of all children with mental retardation and developmental disabilities through age 21. The law was amended in 1986 to guarantee educational services to children with disabilities from age 3 through 21. It provided incentives for states to develop infant and toddler service delivery systems. Additional amendments were authorized and enacted in 1997. Today, most states guarantee intervention services to children with disabilities between birth and 21 years of age. Chapters 4 and 5 present an extended discussion of the importance of the IDEA for parents of children with mental retardation.

The first effective medications for the treatment of mental illness became available in the United States beginning in the mid-1950s and early 1960s. Their use soon became widespread among institutionalized individuals with mental retardation, sometimes to the exclusion of effective non-biological interventions. Unfortunately, medications often were overused and side effects unrecognized. By the 1970s, families began to clamor for less use of "chemical restraints" and more use of educational and behavioral interventions to address the needs of individuals with more severe forms of mental retardation. Their concerns finally prompted federal and state regulatory intervention. As is often the case with ideas and intentions, extreme opinions clashed. By the 1980s, increasingly restrictive and often prohibitive regulations limited the use of psychoactive medications in institutionalized individuals with mental retardation, even when judicious use of medication would have been beneficial. When psychoactive medications were allowed, mandates such as "drug holidays" and annual discontinuation of medications often proved counterproductive.

In the 1990s, newer and safer psychoactive medications became available and psychiatrists became more adept at selecting appropriate target symptoms and dosages (i.e., the lowest dose that was effective, "least effective dose"). As a result, regulatory concerns eased and regulatory agencies adopted more cooperative postures. Care was taken to maintain adequate accountability and to discourage indiscriminate use of psychoactive medications.

During that same decade, families began to demand more community-based services as an alternative to institutional services. Special education programs in public schools expanded from self-contained classrooms to mainstreamed and transitioned school-to-work initiatives. Community living, through group homes or other supported living arrangements, proved that many previously institutionalized individuals could live successfully outside institutions with varying degrees of assistance and structure.

Community work opportunity programs became available to adults with mental retardation. Many were able to move successfully into supported employment in the private sector. Similarly, early intervention programs for preschool-age children with mental retardation proved beneficial neurologically and intellectually, while "retirement" programs for affected senior citizens provided age-appropriate alternatives to institutional care. By the beginning of this century, a number of programs were available for people of all ages. Still, the span of services is not seamless.

Theories of Intelligence and Adaptive Skills

Over the past 100 years educational specialists, theorists, and researchers have attempted to define intelligence. In the process, tests to measure intelligence evolved in the early 20th century and were cited as a more objective method to evaluate individual potential and capability.

In spite of considerable research and debate, no universally accepted definition of intelligence has emerged; different definitions reflect differing perspectives. Wechsler, the designer of the most widely used set of intelligence tests today, defined intelligence as "the aggregate or global capacity of the individual to act purposefully, to think rationally, and to deal effectively with the environment." Other theorists have defined intelligence as the ability to think and reason creatively.

Traditional testing favors verbal capacity as an expression of intelligence. Gardner contends that intelligence is a group of abilities and that testing verbal capacity or ability to calculate is a fragmented approach that does not reveal all aspects of an individual's capabilities. Thus, proponents of so-called "multiple intelligence" theories (such as Gardner) suggest that accurate, complete evaluation provides the means for an individual to demonstrate performance in allied intellectual areas.

In the context of public education services, measuring intelligence by means of conventional tests provides information about a child's capabilities in relation to those of other children of similar age. Tests of intelligence that yield only I.Q. scores do not provide parents or service providers with a fully developed prognosis for any child's learning capacity. Likewise, intelligence and intellectual development are dynamic, changing processes, influenced by environmental experiences, active learning programs, and a host of more complex, individualized factors. Thus, intelligence tests and their administration and interpretation must be considered within the contexts of the child's age, culture, environment, and conditions of testing.

Assessment of Intelligence

Testing methods used by school psychometrists, psychologists, and other diagnosticians are founded on the Binet test (see above). The test was later refined by Lewis Terman of Stanford University (Stanford-Binet test), who developed the instrument termed an "intelligence quotient test" or I.Q. test. With further refinements, this test remains among the most widely used in the United States.

Today's Stanford-Binet instrument uses the concepts of "basal and ceiling ages." The basal age is the point at which an individual passed all test items given. The ceiling age is the point at which that person failed all test items given. Under its precepts, intelligence is normed (that is, standardized within representative age groups whose performance is evaluated in relation to the performance of others) on a bell-shaped curve with a mean (or average) score of 100. An intelligence test standardized with groups who represent only Western cultures would not adequately evaluate the intelligence of a child from a South African culture. A test that has been standardized with children who speak English is not an appropriate measure of intelligence for a child whose native language is Spanish.

Intelligence tests have been criticized as inadequate measures of real world skills. Ecological validity (i.e., the extent to which a test accurately measures an individual's achievements or predicts adult success) is defined by Cole and Gardner as a more relevant standard against which a person's intelligence may be assessed. In truth, intelligence tests are considered to be better predictors of school performance than of basic human intelligence and future success. A child's ability to take and excel on a particular test may only indicate that the child is adept at testing.

Using Intelligence Tests in Educational Settings

Regardless of what intelligence tests measure, they remain a necessary part of determining a child's eligibility for educational supports and other needed services. While many parents and educational theorists find intelligence testing to be an inequitable and inaccurate method for categorizing children, current federal and state regulations still identify children by this means when determining the amount of funds to provide for services.

In determining eligibility for educational supports and other needed services, school psychometrists (those specialists who perform psychological tests) or educational psychologists may use a variety of tests designed to measure innate capabilities to think, reason, and learn. The Wechsler Intelligence Scale for Children, Leiter International Performance Scale, Slosson Intelligence Test, or Stanford-Binet Intelligence Scale may be used for this purpose.

Visual-motor perceptual tests such as the Bender Visual Motor Gestalt Test, Beery Developmental Test of Visual Motor Integration, and Detroit Test of Learning Ability evaluate fine motor skills and sensory perception—that is, how a child uses information received through senses as a means of learning.

Academic skills tests measuring traditional reading, mathematics, and written language skills include the Wechsler Individual Achievement Test and the Woodcock-Johnson Scales of Achievement.

Psychologists may also evaluate children's emotional and behavioral states using tests designed to measure how the children rate their behaviors, attitudes, and feelings at home and at school.

Theories of Adaptive Behavior

Researchers and scientists have described adaptive behavior as clusters of skills. For example, Kamphaus and others have described personal independence (expressed by an individual's skills in self-care, home living, and community independence) as a dimension of adaptive skills. Independent self-care skills such as grooming and dressing are presumed to be related to home living skills needed for household cleaning and food preparation, and for community independence needed for traveling and working.

Responsibility, a second dimension of adaptive behavior, is thought to be expressed in an individual's communication skills, social awareness, and self-management. Receptive and expressive language, social awareness, sexual behavior, personal safety, and time management are considered interrelated skills that demonstrate individual responsibility.

In the decades before the 1960s, individuals were categorized as mildly, moderately, severely, or profoundly retarded based on an I.Q. test score expressed in terms of chronological age. Generally speaking, test results were used to label individuals and to support placement in institutions. As intelligence and I.Q. scores were believed to be fixed throughout life, individuals with severe or profound mental retardation were consigned permanently to custodial care.

In 1964, Parsons State Hospital and Training Center and the American Association on Mental Deficiency (now the American Association on Mental Retardation) received a grant from the National Institute of Mental Health to develop a functional adaptive behavior classification for mental retardation. The resulting Adaptive Behavior Checklist reinforced the concept that individuals could benefit from remedial, prescriptive programs based on levels of adaptive skills more than by simply being labeled through use of intelligence tests.

Researchers and educators sharpened their focus on adaptive skills as educational issues of nondiscriminatory testing and placement, mainstreaming, and normalization emerged during the latter half of the last century. Diagnosing mental retardation now involves much more than testing and labeling. If children take an intelligence test and other capacities are not considered, the testing results provide a narrow, incomplete picture of the individual's capabilities to succeed in living, learning, and working.

Using Adaptive Behavior Tests in Educational Settings

In 1992, the American Association on Mental Retardation refined its definition of mental retardation and included adaptive behavior in ten specific areas of skill: communication, community use, functional academics, health and safety, home living, leisure, self-care, self-direction, social skills, and work.

Comprehensive assessment of adaptive skills implies an evaluation of three domains: practical, conceptual, and social skill functions. When assessing an individual's overall competence, intelligence and adaptive behavior are considered to be demonstrated by performance in the following three areas.

Practical intelligence

Practical skills are demonstrated in activities of daily living, such as self-care skills or occupational skills. Practical intelligence may be regarded as one's ability to maintain and sustain personal independence through the normal activities of daily life. Essential to self-management, practical intelligence is also deemed essential to academics, work, life in the community, and pursuit of leisure interests.

Conceptual intelligence

Conceptual skills are demonstrated in receptive and expressive language, reading, writing, and using money. For example, the recognition of money and its use includes not just identifying coins or correlating the numerical values with purchasing power, but also the "what" and "how" concepts for using money as a means of acquiring goods or as an exchange for property or services. They also demonstrate an understanding of money in its various forms—check, money order, credit card, or currency. They demonstrate understanding that different denominations of coins or currency represent the "how much" conceptualization of using money. Finally, they associate various denominational values with the price of an item or service and comparatively evaluate their resources with an item's price to determine purchasing capacity.

Social intelligence

Social skills are demonstrated in social interrelationships, self-direction, self-control, and participating in group activities. Social intelligence may be regarded as the ability to understand social expectations, others' behavior in relation to oneself, and conduct in keeping with those expectations and situations.

Practical and social intelligence represent those characteristics that most often equate to successful life experiences. When deficiencies are present in one or all of these areas, support services will probably be required.

Maladaptive behaviors—such as aggression, property destruction, self-abusive behaviors, or hyperactivity—represent important considerations when planning educational and support services. Inclusion of maladaptive behaviors within the context of definitions of mental retardation has been questioned by educators, theorists, and researchers. Nevertheless, an individual's maladaptive behaviors usually present support challenges for service providers. Assessment of and program support in response to maladaptive behaviors are components of a comprehensive individualized evaluation process.

Cultural Diversity Issues in Testing

Over the past decades, researchers and educators have grown increasingly concerned about the high percentage of minority students in special education services, particularly individuals diagnosed with intermittent support needs or mild retardation. Many argue that standardized tests may present cultural bias against students who do not come from the English-speaking population and thus can result in an underestimate of intellectual abilities.

Before administering intelligence and achievement tests, test administrators should be familiar with the groups with which the test was standardized, the percentage of minority representation within those groups, and cultural implications for using the test. Test administrators should also consider the preferred language of the individual when selecting and using tests. Home environment, cultural variations, language differences, and cultural perceptions of teachers and other educational specialists should also be evaluated. Failure to consider these factors is likely to bring assessment results into question if the results are used to confirm the presence of a disability.

Evolving Definitions and Classifications of Mental Retardation

The diagnostic elements of mental retardation accepted in the United States by 1900 include onset in childhood, significant intellectual or cognitive limitation, and inability to adapt to the demands of everyday life. In a classification scheme proposed by the American Association on Mental Deficiency, individuals with mental retardation were referred to as "feebleminded" (Committee on Classification, 1910). Three levels of impairment were identified: *idiot*—an individual whose development is arrested at the level of a 2-year-old; *imbecile*—an individual whose development is equivalent to that of a 2- to 7-year-old at maturity; and *moron*—an individual whose mental development is equivalent to that of a 7- to 12-year-old at maturity. These terms are now considered inappropriate and offensive.

During the first half of the twentieth century people diagnosed with mental retardation were considered to be incapable of learning or changing. This limited view has evolved into a more focused, multifaceted perspective that recognizes the dynamic potential of capabilities. Current definitions of mental retardation are based on federal and state regulations, diagnostic criteria developed by clinicians, or a combination of both. Federal and state regulations offer definitions for mental retardation that are used to identify children within a particular educational category for which federal and state funds may then be appropriated.

The Developmental Disabilities Bill of Rights Act of 1978 defined mental retardation and incorporated other developmental disabilities into its legal definition. This definition refers specifically to "developmental disabilities." Within that context, disability is attributed to mental or physical impairments manifested before age 22 years, likely to continue indefinitely, resulting in substantial limitations in three or more specified areas of functioning, and requiring specific and life-long or extended care. In this definition, the term developmental disabilities is considered a broader term than mental retardation and is indicative of more severe, chronic, and medically-oriented states.

The Individuals with Disabilities Education Act (IDEA, 1997) defined mental retardation as "significantly subaverage general intellectual functioning existing concurrently with deficits in adaptive behavior and manifested during the developmental period, that adversely affect a child's educational performance."

Since 1900, the definition of mental retardation has changed at least nine times in the United States. The three clinical definitions of mental retardation commonly used today are similar because their developers tend to coordinate with one another. These definitions all specify both intellectual and adaptive skill deficits as qualifying markers for diagnosing mental retardation.

American association on mental retardation definition

The definition of mental retardation that is gaining greatest
acceptance in the United States is that developed in 1992 by the
American Association on Mental Retardation. According to that
AAMR publication, the I.Q. level below which mental retardation is diagnosed is 70 to 75 (the 5-point variation reflecting
the accuracy of current standard tests of intelligence). The I.Q.
of normal individuals (the majority of people) generally falls
between 80 to 120. Although an "average I.Q." of 100 is commonly quoted, this number has no special significance. It is simply a mathematical term calculated from the total of scores of all
"normal" people tested divided by the number of normal people
tested. In other words, an I.Q. of 100 is a reference point on a
target around which other "normal I.Q. scores" cluster.

The AAMR defines mental retardation as "substantial limitations in present functioning. It is characterized by significantly
subaverage intellectual functioning, existing concurrently with
related limitations in two or more of the following applicable
adaptive skill areas: communication, self-care, home living,
social skills, community use, self-direction, health and safety,
functional academics, leisure and work. Mental retardation
manifests before age 18."

Whereas levels of mental retardation (mild, moderate, severe,
and profound) were formerly diagnosed on the basis of I.Q.,
the 1992 AAMR classification system substituted a system that
defines the support needed in specific areas of functioning and
minimizes reliance on I.Q. measures.

Importantly, the AAMR definition is based on four assumptions considered essential to the meaning of mental retardation.

1. Tests used to determine a valid evaluation and diagnosis
of mental retardation consider the individual's culture and
linguistic diversity as well as communication and behavioral

differences. Failing to consider a child's culture, language used in the home and community, or known performance limitations caused by motor, sensory, or emotional conditions negates test results.

2. When determining deficits in adaptive behavior, deficits in at least two skill areas must be present and identified within the context of the home, community, school, and other environments within which the individual interacts. Due consideration is given to those skills typical of the individual's age peers within those environments.

3. Individuals may have strengths in certain adaptive areas while having deficits in others. A person may demonstrate social competencies but be limited in traditional communication skills.

4. The final assumption represents a working philosophy of support across life stages, asserting that an individual's life functioning will generally improve with directed, sustained supports. This concept suggests that each individual's strengths and needs will guide the choice of strategies to diminish the effects of mental retardation on life functioning and implies that supports, when needed, may be lifelong or intermittent and physical or medical. It also reinforces the notion that ongoing evaluations and support revisions may be both needed and desirable for continued progress. Optimally, supports improve the manner in which an individual meets challenges in daily life, while promoting independence and productivity in the community.

Diagnostic and statistical manual of mental disorders, edition four (DSM-IV-TR) definition

The American Psychiatric Association has produced a classification manual defining mental disorders, among them mental retardation. The DSM-IV-TR is a minor revision of the fourth version of this diagnostic manual. The original DSM-IV was published in 1994; DSM-IV-TR was published in 2000.

Like the AAMR classification system, the DSM-IV-TR bases its diagnosis of mental retardation on a combination of factors: I.Q. of approximately 70 or below on an individually administered, standardized test of intelligence; simultaneous impairments in adaptive functioning in at least two of the defined life areas: communication, self-care, home living, social/interpersonal skills, use of community resources, self-direction, functional academic skills, work, leisure, health, and safety; and onset before age 18 years.

The DSM-IV-TR definition differs from the AAMR definition in that it retains the concept of "levels" of mental retardation.

International statistical classification of diseases and related health problems, 10th revision (ICD-10) definition

ICD-10 is the tenth revision of the International Classification of Diseases (World Health Organization, 1994). It defines mental retardation as a condition of "arrested or incomplete development of the mind" characterized by impaired developmental skills that "contribute to the overall level of intelligence." Impaired developmental skills include language, motor, social, and cognitive (or reasoning and learning) abilities. ICD-10

Table 3.1 DSM-IV Levels of Mental Retardation

Severity	I.Q. Ranges
Mild	50–55 to 70
Moderate	35–40 to 50–55
Severe	20–25 to 35–40
Profound	Below 20–25

notes that adaptive behavior is almost always impaired in people with mental retardation, but the impairment may not be recognized in "protected social environments." Categories are provided for specifying the extent of behavior impairment: none or minimal; significant, requiring treatment or attention; other impairments; no mention of impairments.

According to ICD-10, overall ability, rather than specific impairments, should form the basis for the diagnosis of mental retardation. It holds that levels of intelligence should not be rigidly applied because of problems with the accuracy of testing individuals of one culture with intelligence tests developed in another. Intelligence tests should be standardized according to local cultural norms. If not, ICD-10 suggests that the diagnosis be regarded as "provisional."

According to this international standard, mild mental retardation is diagnosed in individuals who acquire language somewhat late but speak well enough to manage in life. Most are able to take care of themselves although they may develop self-care skills later than normal. Their intellectual disabilities become evident when they attempt to learn to read and write: They can do so, but at a slower pace and to a lesser degree of sophistication. They are capable of earning a living but may have difficulty fulfilling cultural roles, such as coping with marriage or childrearing.

Table 3.2 ICD-10 Levels of Mental Retardation

Severity	I.Q. Range	Mental age (years)
Mild	50–69	9 to <12
Moderate	35–49	6 to <9
Severe	20–34	3 to <6
Profound	Below 20	<3

Moderate mental retardation is diagnosed in individuals who slowly gain limited language skills and are impaired in their ability to care for themselves. Some may learn basic academic skills, do simple work, and engage in social activities. They generally reach their highest level of function only in a structured, supervised setting.

Severe mental retardation is diagnosed in individuals with limited or no language skills and with marked motor or other impairments that point to damage to the central nervous system or to abnormal development.

Profound mental retardation is diagnosed in individuals with severely limited cognitive abilities. They are often bedridden or immobile or severely restricted in their ability to move, incontinent (i.e., lacking bladder and/or bowel control), and unable to provide for their most basic needs.

ICD-10 refers to "mental age," a term derived from intelligence testing that refers to the level at which an individual tested received the same number of correct responses on a standardized I.Q. test as a normal person of the same age. This does not mean that an individual with mental retardation "has the mind of a younger person."

Educational Classifications in Mental Retardation

While medical and psychosocial communities were developing a classification system, so was the educational community. Their three-level system separated school-age children with mental retardation into three groups based on predicted ability to learn (Kirk, Karnes, & Kirk, 1955):

1. Children who were *educable* could learn simple academic skills but not progress above fourth grade level.

2. Children who were *trainable* could learn to care for their daily needs but not many academic skills.
3. Children who were *untrainable* or totally dependent were in need of long term care, possibly in a residential setting.

Some form of this scheme is still in use today in many school systems across the country, although many people consider the scheme to be stigmatizing.

Assessment and Diagnosis of Mental Retardation

The AAMR manual defines a three-step process for diagnosing and classifying mental retardation and emphasizes the need for detailed assessment of individuals and their needs in all relevant aspects of their function, including psychological and emotional status. The process includes the following steps:

1. Administration by a qualified person of one or more standardized intelligence tests and at least one standardized adaptive skills test.
2. Assessment of the individual's strengths and weaknesses in four areas: intellectual and adaptive behavior skills; psychological and emotional considerations; physical, health, and etiological (or causal) factors; and environmental factors. Strengths and weaknesses may be assessed by formal testing, observations, interviews of family members or other key persons in the individual's life, or a combination of those methods.
3. Professionals from various educational backgrounds form an "interdisciplinary" team to determine supportive measures needed to address the identified needs in the four domains noted above. Each supportive measure is assigned

Table 3.3 Levels of supportive measures

Intermittent	Measures that will be used on an "as needed basis"— may be needed by an individual periodically over the life span, but not on a daily or routine basis; e.g., assistance in finding a new job
Limited	Measures that may be needed over a limited time span; e.g., assistance in completing school and transitioning into a work or job training situation
Extensive	Measures providing assistance in a specific life area on a daily basis without time limitation, and in home or work environments
Pervasive	Measures that are constantly (daily) required across all environmental and life areas and may include life-sustaining measure

one of four basic levels of intensity—intermittent, limited, extensive, and pervasive.

Other Developmental Disabilities

Mental retardation is one form of developmental disability. Legislation regarding developmental disabilities was first introduced as part of congressional action in 1963. In 1990, Congress reauthorized Public Law 101-496, The Developmental Disabilities Assistance and Bill of Rights Act, that included the following definition: "The term 'developmental disability' means a severe, chronic disability of a person 5 years of age or older which is attributable to a mental or physical impairment or combination of mental and physical impairments; is manifested before the person attains age 22; is likely to continue indefinitely; results in substantial functional limitations in three or more of the following areas of major life activity: self-care, receptive and expressive language, learning, mobility, self-direction, capacity for independent living and economic self-sufficiency; reflects the person's need for a combination and sequence of special interdisciplinary or generic care, treatment or other services which are of lifelong or extended duration and are individually planned and coordinated."

The term "developmental delay" is used when a child does not demonstrate growth and development normal for the child's age. The delays may be present in only one area or in several. For example, a child may be walking at the age expected but not using language within the expected age ranges. Developmental delays may occur with other medical conditions or when a child's home environment does not provide stimulation sufficient to promote optimum social, language, motor, or sensory growth. The term also may be applied to children when their age may make definite diagnosis of mental retardation inaccurate or inappropriate given their limited performance on available individualized standardized tests or other assessment methods. In the absence of clear and significant subaverage deficits in both intellectual ability and adaptive skills, a diagnosis of mental retardation is both premature and possibly stigmatizing.

While children with developmental delays may not have mental retardation, the delays should not be treated as insignificant. Some children may overcome such delays, but parents and physicians cannot rely on waiting to allow the child time to recover delayed skills. Delayed development may predict lifelong challenges. Waiting may allow delays to become more critical. Determining the source of the problems and beginning any needed testing and interventions as soon as possible may minimize difficulties as the child grows older.

4. The First Six Years: Infants, Toddlers, and Preschool Children

Life's early years are critical. A baby or young child is the precursor of the adult. A lifetime's aspirations, nurtured during pregnancy, come into focus during a child's first years. Childhood, particularly the first six years, is the most critical, irreplaceable time for closing gaps left by disabilities or delays. Early intervention is vital to diminish those effects.

Legislation, Regulation, and Policy

Prior to 1975, states faced few, if any, federal mandates for educational services. Specialized supports were limited. With meager services, families either educated their children at home or chose out-of-home residential placement. Years of disregard and unconcern slowly galvanized parent and advocacy organizations to a grassroots resolve for change in how children were treated. Largely through their individual and collective presence in legislative and policy-making forums, citizens gained support for substantive reforms.

Eventually, Congress established new directions that became the basis for unprecedented federal and state modifications. The most important of these are summarized in Appendix C. In many respects, recent laws—such as The Americans with

Disabilities Act of 1990—gained momentum from the citizen-directed disability movement now active in the United States.

In 1975 Congress passed the Education for All Handicapped Children Act, regarded by many authorities as setting the foundation for today's disability rights principles. This and subsequent re-authorizations mandated educational services for children from birth through 21 years of age.

In 1997 Congress passed the Individuals with Disabilities Education Act (IDEA), landmark legislation that defined the rights of U.S. citizens with a wide range of medical disabilities, including mental retardation. The Act defines "child with a disability" as one who has been evaluated according to prescribed guidelines, has been found to have a disability in one or more specifically defined areas, and has need of special education and related services. The Act recognizes 13 categories of disabilities eligible for special services: autism, deafness, deaf-blindness, hearing impairment, mental retardation, multiple disabilities, orthopedic impairment, other health impairment, serious emotional disturbance, specific learning disability, speech or language impairment, traumatic brain injury, and visual impairment.

Under IDEA, each state is required to submit a plan that describes how its educational services will comply with the law. A state's department of education is generally recognized as the designated agency for children from three years of age through 21 years. However, services for children from birth through three years of age may be provided by a state department of health or another agency. An informational parent's handbook about special education laws and regulations may be obtained by contacting the state's department of education, office of special education.

While local education agencies may have minor variations in evaluation and service planning, all are required to adhere to six provisions of the IDEA:

• All children will receive a free, appropriate public education. State and school districts have the responsibility of paying for an education even if services are provided in another setting.

• Parents and children are guaranteed the right of due process. Acting as the child's advocate, parents and families have both the right and the responsibility to become and remain involved in creating a plan that strengthens an individual's skills and supports needs.

• Parents have the right to challenge and appeal any decision throughout the process, including identification, evaluation, placement, and ongoing evaluation of their child.

• Each child will receive a non-biased, multidisciplinary evaluation as a basis for eligibility determination. Tests must be selected that accurately reveal both strengths and weaknesses.

• Each child will receive services that are described in an Individualized Education Plan (IEP). The plan must be based on test results and developed with the child's family and educational team. Related services such as speech-language therapy, occupational or physical therapy, or other supports must be specified in the IEP. Infants, toddlers and pre-school aged children receive services described in an Individual Family Service Plan, or IFSP.

• Children will be educated in their least restrictive environment (LRE), that is, educated with peers who are not disabled to the maximum extent feasible. Services in separate, self-contained settings are deemed appropriate only when the nature or severity of disabilities prohibit inclusion in the least restrictive environment.

The IDEA contains specific procedural safeguards for eligible children and their families. Procedural safeguards are rights that ensure federal and state protections and mechanisms for resolving or mediating disputes; for example, the right to accept or decline any early intervention services without jeopardizing eligibility for other early intervention services. For a complete list of rights under IDEA, refer to Appendix C.

Finding Early Intervention Services and Supports

When parents sense that their child is having difficulties, learning about the evaluation and placement process may not be so intimidating. At such times, parents may have already taken the first step in contacting physicians or state health or education providers about suspected disabilities.

If parents have little or no experience with these processes, their first contact with health care and educators may cause alarm. Unfamiliarity with procedures, parental rights, the child's rights or how to begin only contributes to apprehension. Regardless of what parents eventually decide, getting more information as soon as possible restores a valuable sense of control and advocacy for their child.

No two children develop in the same way or at the same rate. Children demonstrate learning differences for many reasons, not all attributable to disabilities. A developmental milestone is a skill or behavior that a child tends to use at a particular age. Infants, toddlers, and preschool-age children can be expected to attain these milestones at given ages (see Appendix B). If a child is not attaining the milestones or has apparent difficulties in mastering skills, a comprehensive assessment will reveal more.

Evaluation determines if a child is eligible for services. In the context of an individual's community, cultural background, and language, evaluations are be useful in service planning. Other considerations are of equal importance. The presence or absence of known factors may dictate different evaluation and assessment strategies. For example, some infants have conditions that suggest mental retardation or developmental delay, such as Down syndrome. Other children may lack obvious physical markers but be at risk for disability. In such cases, evaluation may reveal conditions that predispose a child to disability.

In either case, parents, professionals, and physicians are rightfully cautious about applying too-specific diagnoses for children under the age of three years. An infant or toddler presents different assessment questions from those posed for a child who is first tested during elementary school years. Regardless of a child's age, suspected disability, or risk for disability, it is crucial to remember that test results obtained during the first six years are not necessarily indicative of his or her potential.

Parents may feel angry, afraid, frustrated, and overwhelmed— emotions that are not resolved quickly. Having a child with special needs means that parents must refocus on a different future and shift their energies to overcoming the disability's effects. Understandably, this responsibility may seem beyond their reach at times. New parents may find that support groups offer opportunities to talk with people who have similar emotional and practical challenges.

Parents are the most important individuals in their children's lives and know their children better than any service provider. If a team is to function optimally, parents must get involved and remain committed throughout a child's early years. IDEA recognizes that parents have important roles in working with physicians, teachers, therapists, and other specialists to create meaningful programs. As their child's most significant advocates, they must be informed about and responsive to the child's needs and active in the decision-making process.

Assessing Infants, Toddlers and School-aged Children

Developing comprehensive understanding of children requires time, careful evaluation strategies, sensitive testing by a knowledgeable, professional team, and thoughtful interpretation of results. Assessment includes information about the environment and conditions within which children live and learn—at home or elsewhere. The collected information offers valuable clues as to how children communicate, take care of themselves, or travel in their environment. Assessment identifies sources of possible disability, reveals factors that may have a bearing on performance, and provides information needed for the development of individualized family service plans as well as methods to measure progress over time.

Parents' assessment questions will change over time, though most concerns focus on getting useful information that makes a difference in their children's lives.

- How can I find out if my baby has a disability?
- What kind of disability does my baby have?
- Who will help me find what I need?
- How can I be certain that my toddler's needs are being met?
- What will happen to my child when he begins school?
- What kind of life can my child expect as an adult?

Providing Early Intervention Services

IDEA recognizes "children with special needs" as children
with disabilities or children at risk for disabilities and mandates services for eligible individuals. States must provide early
intervention services for children with disabilities, ages birth
to three years. From ages three through five years, children
receive special education programs and related services.

When a family-directed, multidisciplinary evaluation con-
cludes that a child is eligible, services must be provided by
people who are qualified to work with children within these
age ranges. States are mandated to assign a service coordinator
who helps families find needed services, interpret requirements,
and assist with evaluation, placement, and educational processes.
The service coordinator will assist the family while the child
receives services and during transition to preschool. Many
resources are available to "decode" medical, therapeutic, or
educational terms (see Appendix D).

Service providers are required to develop a written, individualized family service plan that will be reviewed with the family every six months and evaluated each year for its continued
appropriateness. The state is required to fully explain the plan's
contents and must obtain informed written consent prior to
providing services. If parents do not approve of a particular portion or aspect of services, the state is then required to provide
services for which consent is obtained.

Person-centered Planning: The Sooner, The Better

No one is considered incapable of learning or becoming a
member of a community. Transition planning (i.e., planning
for life needs) is a reasonable outcome of individualized services.

Planning for education, independent living, and economic self-sufficiency will help in the realization of life goals in living, learning, and working. The individual is both the focus of the process and its directing influence. Within a collaborative framework, the individual and the team talk about individual life goals. Capabilities are emphasized. Disabilities are acknowledged but not regarded as impediments.

Working with Service and Support Specialists

Federal law requires comprehensive multidisciplinary evaluations of physical health, vision, hearing, medical status, cognitive development, communication, social and emotional status, and adaptive development. Consent for evaluations is called "informed consent"; that is, a child may not be tested without the parents' full understanding of the evaluation's intent and proposed use of results. Prior to first-time testing, parents must give written approval. The team must provide detailed information about reasons for testing, type of tests proposed, and purpose of tests, enabling parents to decide what is in the child's best interests.

Trained individuals must administer and interpret tests and glean information from all available resources before attempting a specific diagnosis. Determining the child's present functioning capabilities is central to valid interpretations and comparisons. Accordingly, tests evaluate the child's reactions in social or learning situations, emotional behavioral qualities, and other skills that influence learning. Speech-language pathologists, audiologists, physical or occupational therapists, counselors, or medical specialists may be on the team. A psychologist, psychiatrist, psychometrist, or other behavioral specialist team member observes a child interacting in as many living and learning environments as possible. Physicians will compile the child's medical and family histories, examining developmental milestones and other medical information. Hearing, vision, speech, language, central nervous system functioning, and motor skills will be evaluated. People who are significant in the child's life should be interviewed.

Infants and young children may present age-related fears during test sessions. They may be apprehensive in the presence of unfamiliar people or concerned about being separated from their parent in a strange setting. A parent can ease anxieties by sharing information about the conditions that create the greatest comfort. For infants, the mother's presence is generally reassuring. For older children, parents may explain as much as they believe their child can understand and remain present during unfamiliar procedures.

Throughout the process, parents should participate actively. Monitoring the evaluation progress, attending scheduled meetings, and answering any questions from the child will support the total partnership. Parents find it helpful to record vital information, questions, answers and other resources. Maintaining contact files with individuals' names and telephone numbers is useful for future reference.

Working with Physicians and Other Health Care Professionals

Medical practitioners, among the first professionals to be acquainted with a family, hold a preeminent role in supporting families. Obstetricians and gynecologists are among the more important practitioners positioned to advocate for genetic counseling, early and adequate prenatal care and nutrition, and evaluative studies in cases of suspected high risk pregnancies. As an ethical consideration, these professionals have an inherent responsibility to provide expectant mothers with prompt, informed advice relative to her unborn child's ultimate welfare, health, and life experiences.

Evaluative techniques such as amniocentesis, urinalysis, ultrasound, and blood screening can now be expanded with 3-D ultrasound tests. No more complicated than traditional ultrasound, this new methodology creates a lifelike image of the developing fetus, providing medical specialists and expectant parents with a near-birth quality photograph. Typically done between the 22nd and 36th weeks of pregnancy, this technology prepares a parent and family for the birth of a child with observable disabilities.

Certain physical or chromosomal disabilities are observable at or before birth; other disabilities are more difficult to detect. Because early detection is so important, all states require newborn screening for certain conditions. While the newborn is in the delivery suite, a blood sample is taken from the child's heel and deposited on filter paper for laboratory examination. The results may reveal conditions that, if left untreated, result in mental retardation. Unfortunately, screening for metabolic disorders and other conditions that are difficult to detect is not consistent from one state to the next.

Recently introduced newborn screening techniques provide information about the possible presence of many conditions. A new procedure, tandem mass spectrometry, supplements routine blood sampling taken from the newborn's heel. While traditional blood sampling tests for three to ten disorders, this technique may detect up to 25 metabolic disorders, including phenylketonuria. It also identifies infants at risk from organic acid and fatty acid oxidation disorders, which can result in disability or death if left untreated. While not yet widely available, this procedure represents the next generation of newborn screening instruments.

According to the American Academy of Family Physicians (AAFP), follow-up care of infants at risk for retardation and other developmental disabilities includes regular screening and monitoring as soon as one week after discharge and continuing through the first year of life. The AAFP notes that 10–20% of infants with a birth weight under 1,500 grams (three pounds, five ounces) have developmental disabilities. While these physical conditions in infants and children are not, in and of themselves, suggestive of disabilities, medical experts advise that evidence of a single developmental abnormality should trigger additional evaluations.

A physician who suspects developmental delays or disabilities should refer parents to the appropriate state contact. With parental permission, the physician may also wish to initiate contact, ensuring prompt referral.

The State Children's Health Insurance Program (SCHIP)

Important new federal legislation now provides health insurance for children through age 18 years. The SCHIP was passed as part of the Balanced Budget Act of 1997. A new mandated partnership between federal and state governments, SCHIP established a five-year, $24 billion fund for uninsured American children. SCHIP is targeted toward families with incomes too high for Medicaid eligibility and too low for affordable health insurance. Funds may not be used to supplement existing health insurance.

Information Resources for Parents

Information is available from each state's designated lead agency. In some states the lead agency will be their state education agency; in others, the state health and human services agency will be designated. Government agencies with contact numbers are listed in the governmental section of telephone directories or can be located through directory assistance.

All states and territories maintain a federally-mandated protection and advocacy system as required by the Protection and Advocacy for Persons with Developmental Disabilities (PADD) Program. This system provides legal, administrative, and other appropriate remedies to protect and promote rights of people with developmental disabilities. (Additional information about this and other consumer resources is listed in Appendix D.)

5. School-Aged Children, Adolescents, and Teenagers

A child's life from 5 to 18 years is a busy, challenging period. During adolescence, as Erik Erikson noted, young people focus on school and friends. They learn to work productively and independently while seeking their unique identity. Though these years may be more difficult for people with disabilities, appropriate supports may "level the playing field."

The IDEA: What the Law Means During School Years

Public Law 105-17, the Individuals with Disabilities Education Act of 1997 (IDEA), applies to children of school age, adolescents, and teenaged youth. The act defines participation with peers who are not disabled and requires modified practices to achieve "education in the general curriculum."

In this age group, the individualized education program (IEP) must explain how education will be modified for a student's participation with students in the general program and must define necessary special accommodations or modifications. General classroom inclusion may be inappropriate, but when this is the case, the IEP team must support its conclusion, describing why a student will not be in the general curriculum or in regular extracurricular or non-academic activities.

Parents must be included in the decision-making processes of both initial testing and periodic reevaluations in later years and must receive written notice prior to beginning any exploration of special needs. Parents should know that their informed written consent is required for both the initial evaluation and reevaluations and again separately for placement permission. Reevaluations must be conducted not less than once every three years, when educational conditions warrant, or if parents or teachers request retesting.

Information from a variety of tests and sources is used to determine if a disability is present and the most appropriate education for the student. Multidisciplinary team members include parents of the child, special education teachers, general education teachers, and specialists such as psychologists, speech-language pathologists, or other support personnel. When the evaluation is finished, a copy of the evaluation report and eligibility determination documents must be provided to the parents.

Special Rule for Eligibility Determination

In its revisions to the IDEA, Congress cited statistics that indicated substantial numbers of children have been mislabeled as "disabled." The "rule for eligibility determination" now requires that the evaluation team and parents consider whether a child's actual educational difficulties are the result of a disability rather than factors unrelated to disabilities, such as poor academic preparation, use of languages other than English, or inadequate instruction.

Active Partnering: Being an Effective Advocate

An "advocate" is a person who assists or supports another individual. To be effective advocates, parents need time and energy to learn about federal and state laws, state plan requirements, and other related legal and educational rights. Active partnering with the local agency and team requires honest discussions about a child's life span expectations and needs. This partnership implies equal measures of assertiveness, communication, and shared responsibilities. As with any partnership, parents and educators may encounter intermittent challenges but should maintain working, non-threatening relationships with one another.

How Parents Can Help Their Child Understand Testing

Parents can help their children understand "being tested" and what they will learn from this process. Children may be reassured to know that teachers and other people who will talk with them are all interested in helping them in school. Parents should explain that there will be different tests that will help teachers understand more about how the child learns. Children should be allowed to express fears or ask questions.

Parents need to be informed about how proposed tests will be used to answer specific questions. As with younger children, parents should advise evaluators of their children's past performance, preferred learning strategies, and any specific accommodations needed during the assessment. Parents should also monitor the assessment's progress.

While states' plans vary, the evaluation typically explores five areas of learning and development: education, medical, social, psychological status, and related areas such as sensory and communication capacities. Educational skills will be tested. Individualized, standardized tests should explore all areas of the child's suspected disability. School performance records may demonstrate patterns or trends evident in the academic history or other events occurring simultaneously with performance changes. Current classroom performance and rate of learning should be examined in conjunction with curriculum requirements. Most sessions include psychological evaluation; that is, how children react in social or learning situations, their emotional and behavioral qualities, and other skills that influence learning.

Classroom observation and interviews of people significant to the child should be included in the assessment. With the assistance of parents, medical and social histories will be compiled, examining developmental milestones and other health information. Hearing and vision acuity, speech, language, central nervous system functioning, or motor skills will be assessed.

What IDEA Says about Assistive Technology (AT)

IDEA requires consideration of possible assistive technology needs for all children affected by its mandates. Federal laws define "assistive technology" as "any piece of equipment or product system, whether acquired commercially off the shelf, modified or customized, that is used to increase, maintain or improve functional capabilities of the individual with disabilities."

Assistive technology can offer new experiences for students who may be limited in their ability to control their environment, participate in class, or communicate basic needs and wants. A wide range of devices is available and, although not necessarily expensive, parents and professional educators alike may find costs and the rapidly changing market to be challenging. Selecting, finding, funding, and maintaining the most compatible devices can be complicated.

Parents and educators must research different types of equipment and analyze design features to make informed acquisitions. Their decisions should be based on comprehensive evaluations that match students with the most appropriate devices. As parents consider particular technological aids, answering the following five basic questions may ensure appropriate selection and use of AT.

How is AT used in educational settings?

Assistive technology connects people with their environments. Communication and control of one's life are essential elements to quality of life. The ability to communicate is the single greatest predictor of educational success. Assistive technologies advance these abilities.

Beginning in infancy, children learn through play. Using an adaptive switch to manipulate a battery-operated toy, toddlers learn that their actions can control part of their environment. As children move to the classroom, adaptive learning tools replace earlier assistive toys.

The decision to obtain and use assistive technology is best determined by the individual, the individual's parents, and other team members. Over the past decade, educators and specialists have realized that AT is more than computers, printers, and software. Today, students are making great strides through simple modifications to traditional toys, hardware, software, and materials.

How is the AT evaluation conducted?

Before testing, parents and the team may consider the child's age, use of the evaluation results, and desired goals. During the evaluation, the evaluator will determine if a child has consistent, demonstrated skills to use technology. Observing the child's performance on certain tasks, the evaluator can determine preferred equipment uses. The evaluator may also consider non-educational uses and the relative cost of equipment when compared to learning goals.

What information may be gained from the evaluation?

Parents and educators want to know if a child has consistent, reliably demonstrated skills that may be used with specific devices. Given the relative importance of communication and environmental control, some AT proponents believe that any individual can and should use technology even though that person may not demonstrate consistent use of requisite skills.

The evaluation helps identify which general device category may be the most appropriate match for the individual's learning style. It may be necessary to extend the evaluation process over several sessions, focusing on different information needs. The team may then determine that certain aid categories will convey more accurately the student's true capabilities, strengths, needs and methods for using specific devices with the student's IEP.

After the IEP is developed, the team will be better informed about choosing from among available devices in a particular category. The selected device should enable the student to maximize learning potential in the five core learning areas and have a broad range of educational applications. For example, students with visual deficits may benefit from sensory enhancers, such as Braille writers, with input and output capabilities. If unable to use a traditional computer keyboard, a student may use modified touch-sensitive pads or touch screens. Students with limited cognitive skills, restricted range of motion, or other physical challenges may use equipment or hardware with adaptive switches, amplifiers, or other environmental control devices.

How can the team find the most appropriate technology devices and supports?

Today, a virtually limitless resource network exists to both inform and support parents and team members in finding, funding, and maintaining technological aids and devices. Availability varies from state to state, and new resources emerge on a regular basis. Given the vast market, making a knowledgeable selection of one suitable product from among hundreds can be challenging.

Under broadened federal accessibility regulations, system developers have expanded both products and marketing strategies in schools, public buildings, transportation providers, and workplaces. Educational and therapeutic organizations, universities, research centers, advocacy groups, parent groups, and other allied agencies also have increased available information and support.

Successful efforts have one common theme—commitment. Parents and their support network make an initial commitment to research and understand the rapidly evolving AT field, asking questions, keeping information files—in short, developing step-by-step plans to obtain devices. This process ensures that aids meet and maintain intended educational uses as a student's needs change over time.

The Internet is an invaluable research tool, although web sites vary in content, scope, and usefulness. If parents do not have home computer access, they may have access through community libraries or public school libraries. Information may be found in sites for state and federal governmental agencies, university research centers, grant projects, parent/advocacy organizations, or professional general or special education associations. Generally, these web sites post links to related information sites.

Closing the Gap is a website that focuses on educational needs. Founded by parents of an individual who is deaf, Closing the Gap provides information on computer technology in special education and rehabilitation. Its site map contains a bookmark collection, resource directory, library, calendar of events, conference information, question and answer, and classified sections.

The Trace Research and Development Center, College of Engineering, University of Wisconsin at Madison website contains information for all students and individuals. Founded in 1971, the Trace Center was organized to help people who are non-speaking and who have severe disabilities. This site requires greater technical expertise, providing a list of support resources for product modification. Resources are organized by general topic, disability type, assessment and evaluation services, and product type. Information is also categorized by disability resources and organizations, accessible design organizations, chat rooms, forums, funding sources and government research.

How can parents locate and pay for technology learning aids?

In many instances, families either pay for AT or seek assistance from organizations or groups. Some vendors or product manufacturers may donate equipment and should be considered as possible resources.

Among children who are eligible for Medicaid funds, roughly half of families receive third-party financial help. Public funding varies. States do not use the same categorical definitions and differ in equipment for which funds are available. As a requirement of its Medicaid plan, each state defines eligible equipment. Generally speaking, AT tends to be categorized as durable medical equipment, prosthetic or orthotic equipment, or medical supplies.

As with other federal programs, Medicaid regulations, guidelines, and application procedures change from time to time. Parents are advised to consult with their local office of the Social Security Administration or state Medicaid authority to determine specific application procedures for equipment, devices, or aids.

States are now recognizing alternative and augmentative communication (AAC) devices under "medically necessary equipment." In most instances, these devices meet the Medicaid-recognized definition of "durable medical equipment." AAC devices may also be regarded as prosthetic equipment. Under federally defined speech therapy services, such equipment is likely applicable as "necessary supplies and equipment." If the device is the only means of communication with others, the product should be a recognized benefit under the Medicaid program.

In large measure, an individual's physician is regarded as the professional responsible for making the determination of medical necessity. Parents should be certain that their physician is fully informed of the specific Medicaid and state requirements that govern medical necessity. The physician's statements with regard to medical necessity must be accurate, stated in correct terminology, complete, and sufficiently detailed to enable the Medicaid reviewer to make a determination for approval. States require that families obtain written authorization and approval before buying any allowable equipment. Parents should not order or purchase products without prior written Medicaid authorization and should not allow any unauthorized person to make unapproved purchases.

Individualized Education Planning: Learning for Living and Working

Under IDEA, the IEP team of school-age children consists of a general education teacher, a special education teacher, an agency representative who supervises special education services and has knowledge of the general curricular program, other people invited by the agency, the parents, and the student (as appropriate to capabilities). For students at least 14 years old, the team will also include agency representatives providing transition-to-work activities. Transition activities must be provided, as appropriate, for students 16 years old or younger.

The IEP details goals and objectives so that any reader gains a clear picture of the student and the student's present performance levels. Goals should be based on what the student needs to learn; how, when, and where instruction will be provided; how long and with what frequency instruction will be provided; and how progress will be measured. The plan should describe how the student communicates, cares for personal needs, any behaviors that may hinder learning and hearing, vision, and motor skills. If a student uses a communication board to express himself, the IEP should include information about the device, the student's preferred method of using the board, and other relevant details. If a student has behavioral difficulties that interfere with learning, the IEP should identify the behaviors and the methods teachers should use to respond and to prevent behavioral influences. If a student is blind, deaf, or has cerebral palsy or other physical challenges, the IEP must provide specific instructional guidance for meeting the student's needs in relation to those factors.

Transition from School to Work

When Congress revised the IDEA, it strengthened requirements for preparation for work beyond traditional school years. Research indicated that a large percentage of students lacked marketable work skills. Students often received no additional training after completing their school requirements. If provided, training was too general and typically offered only during the final twelve months' education. Such inadequate planning often left young men and women without productive daily activities, employable skills, or future usefulness.

Ideally, transition planning begins early enough to provide a student with meaningful opportunities to explore the working world. Transition identifies services for employment and adult living, such as placing the student at a potential work site with a job coach for a specified number of hours per week.

Students may have unrealistic hopes about who they are and how they will be part of their community. Disabled or not, many young people have difficulty in making a clear choice of how they want to spend their adult years. Transition planning helps students by providing them with hands-on opportunities to see what a job may be like before making life goal decisions and focuses on the student's future vision:

- Where does the student see himself after finishing his educational program?
- Is the student interested in gainful employment?
- What kind of job?
- What skills does the student now have that can be used on the job?
- What skills may be needed in the future?
- What agency or agencies will be responsible for working with the student, paying for transition services or related supports?

Obviously, competitive employment may not be a viable option for young people with pervasive communicative, medical or physical needs. While these students may participate minimally in transition planning, the team should identify essential life goals that accentuate strengths and address ongoing needs.

Congress also addressed a student's age of majority and transfer of rights while transition services are planned. In some states, a student's rights transfer from the parents to the student at the age of majority, that is, the age at which the student is regarded as an independent adult. Under applicable conditions, the IEP must state that the student has been advised of transfer rights at least one year before the student reaches majority age.

What IDEA Requires for Disciplining Students with Disabilities

Revised discipline guidelines present challenges for parents and educators alike. In brief, that portion of the law is referenced under "Placement in Alternative Educational Setting" as ten separate, interdependent guidelines. IDEA details specific procedures for the local educational authority (LEA) if a student brings a weapon to school, or has, sells, solicits for sale, or uses illicit drugs while at school. Under such circumstances, the law requires that the LEA determine whether or not the action was a function of the student's disability. The law defines actions for behavioral evaluation, parent notification, student suspension, time frames for actions, alternative placements, and procedures for appeals and hearings.

Life Education: Growing Up Is More Than Books

As children develop, self-awareness takes on different perspectives in relation to others. Being popular and liked is important for children, adolescents, and adults. Young people become more curious about how others regard them. Girls and boys become aware of their attractiveness to others and their ability to establish and maintain friendships. Sexual interests emerge. Helping young people balance the social and sexual aspects of life is essential to healthy adult relationships.

Parents may have difficulty counseling their children with developmental disabilities about interpersonal relationships. While parents may accept and view sexuality as a life process, accepting their child as a person with developing sexual feelings may not be as simple. Parents should remember that ignoring that aspect of their children's needs will not diminish its influence. They must come to see "the child" as "a consenting adult," an emotional dilemma that confronts both natural protectiveness and, perhaps, a larger inability to reconcile perceived disparities between disability and human sexuality. When someone has mental retardation but is legally regarded as a consenting adult, parents may find talk about sexual issues unreasonable, disturbing, or offensive. In truth, mature interpersonal relationships may not be a probable life goal for every person with a disability. For example, individuals with pervasive medical or cognitive needs may have little expectation of sexual relations, dating, or marriage.

As young people with retardation become interested in being part of a group, new opportunities may arise for activities outside the home. Certain social skills are expected, including knowing how to act in a friend's home and in restaurants or theaters, how to enjoy conversations, being part of a group, learning about friendships, and appropriate social behaviors with friends of the opposite sex. These skills emerge more naturally with opportunities to feel comfortable and natural in social activities.

Parents can prepare their children to enjoy these occasions by including them in family outings at an early age. Children learn about relationships from watching adults. Parents, parents of friends, and other adult individuals act and talk in certain ways toward each other. These cues, both verbal and non-verbal, are different among cultures, communities, and sexes. For example, a woman may not talk with or act toward a man in the manner that she interacts with another woman. Likewise, adults do not treat children as they treat other adults. The ability to use social cues skillfully is learned over time in different settings and contexts with different people.

As children grow older, non-family relationships become important. Friendships may eventually result in a more selective "pairing". A young person, regardless of the presence of a disability, may want such a relationship. Parents should be prepared by providing guidance about dating relationships, how to act while on a date, and appropriate types of physical contact in public settings.

Sharing Information about Birth Control and Sexually Transmitted Diseases

Responsible parenting includes honest, open communication about sex in terms that the young person can understand. All young people who demonstrate interest in members of the opposite sex need to be supported with information about birth control and sexually transmitted diseases. Ignoring the possibility of an unexpected pregnancy or exposure to disease is neither responsible nor practical. Isolating children with mental retardation from desired outings and activities is not a reasonable solution or prevention tactic.

At some point, responsible parenting means changing from oversight, presence, and guidance to teaching by example. Young people—particularly those with mental retardation— must be given information, skills, and experiences and then allowed to exercise decision-making that promotes independence and self-protection.

Considering Longer-term Relationships

Longer-term relationships should not be an expectation for every young person. When marriage is a life desire, parents should help their maturing child find and understand information about being married, marriage responsibilities, couple relationships, establishing and maintaining a home, dual-career relationships, and family planning. Pre-marriage workshops, seminars, and counseling services are available for couples with retardation who are interested in establishing a longer-term relationship.

Whether or not a couple establishes a legally-recognized marital relationship, a man and woman with mental retardation who are living as a couple should be assisted in getting genetic counseling prior to considering pregnancy. A primary health care provider, physician, or local health department can provide information about necessary medical tests and help understanding the results. Other information resources are accessible through the Internet by searching topics such as "genetic counseling," "genetic screening," or "family planning."

Recognizing Other Social and Sexual Development Concern

Certain social and sexual behaviors are considered not appropriate in most cultures. Most people find it unacceptable to expose one's body, masturbate, or fondle another individual in public. Parents may find it necessary to confront these behaviors. During early years, children should be guided without parental overreacting. Overreaction may create feelings of shame or heighten interest in a parent's reaction.

Often a primary concern, masturbation may have certain religious or moral implications from a parent's own upbringing.

Among earlier generations, masturbation was taboo, typically regarded as "not normal," "perverted," or "deviant." With today's different attitudes about self-gratification and physical release, this practice is more accepted for both sexes.

Parents may find it necessary to provide guidance about masturbation in the appropriate place and time. While the behavior itself is natural, the ability to know when and where to masturbate is not always understood. Again, parents are cautioned against overreaction. For a young person who understands verbal instruction or guidance, simply saying, "Go to your room and close the door" may be sufficient. A person with profound or pervasive cognitive deficits may not fully understand explanations. Behavioral shaping may be more effective—that is, interrupting the behavior and taking the person to a private setting.

Being an Adult Is More Than Sexuality

All parents wish to protect their children. Parents of children with disabilities probably shield them with greater vigilance, imagining the child's vulnerability in adult life. Any child who is unprepared and uneducated about life is vulnerable, regardless of whether that child has a disability. Young people need guidance from adults whom they trust and respect. Parents may struggle with the idea of their children living independently given real and imagined fears about 21st century hazards. Life questions include:

- How will they manage a job?
- How will they manage finances?
- What will happen to them if I cannot be with them?
- How will they make decisions if they cannot ask me what to do?
- What if they are injured in an accident?

Parents have an overarching responsibility to help their children become as independent as possible. This means teaching them about taking care of their own needs, learning about social relationships, getting along with co-workers, developing and being friends, being part of a community or group, and finding recreation. Independence also means being able to protect oneself, to recognize potentially harmful situations, and to know and communicate one's boundaries both verbally and non-verbally. Successful use of these skills reduces a young person's vulnerabilities and improves self-reliance and self-concept.

Education for Personal Protection

Research indicates that individuals with mental retardation disproportionately tend to be victims of sexual abuse. Sexual abuse may occur at any place and any time. Education is a primary means of protecting self against unwanted sexual contact. Young people need to know the difference between desired sexual relations and unwanted abuse. They need to be taught what sexual abuse is, how they can tell someone if they have been abused or threatened, what words to use, and which trusted adults they can go to for protection and support.

Informed Consent: Sexual Rights Versus Protection from Harm

United States constitutional rights and general laws for individuals with disabilities apply with equal vigor to individuals with mental retardation. Within a legal context, individuals with mental retardation have certain rights to sexual expression that are further defined within a context of "informed consent."

Informed consent is generally considered as an individual's decision-making capacity when provided information and asked to select an action from options, as well as the ability to understand the consequences of that choice. Applying this concept to sexual rights is a complicated issue. Basically, United States law provides for personal decisions about sexual activity, marriage, having children, or using birth control. Additionally, states have different laws with regard to acceptable practices among consenting individuals of legally recognized adult age and protection from being coerced into harmful, unwanted sexual contact.

The American Association on Mental Retardation (AAMR) publication *A Guide to Consent* addresses legal and ethical issues of major life areas of self-determination, including sexual activity. Written largely as a professional policy and program guideline, this publication provides essential benchmarks, or guidelines, to support and assist people with mental retardation.

Informed consent for sexual activity implies the person's knowledge and understanding of the act, its possible consequences, and its voluntary nature. The AAMR consent publication has a chapter that offers legal and clinical guidelines for parents, physicians, or counselors when talking about this aspect of life.

6. The Adult Years

As people become more independent, meaningful parental support need not be relinquished. Parents, siblings, family, and friends may be lifelong sources of friendship, counsel, and aid. This becomes more important to those with mental retardation. This chapter speaks to needs and concerns of mentally retarded adults.

Over the first 18 years, people mature gradually. Some gain skills with little or minimal difficulty. Others advance in certain areas but may lag in others. In truth, few people are ready to assume every adult right or responsibility as they reach the age of majority. Through a network of significant people, a young adult finds a ready reserve of guidance, legal information, and friendly assistance to close lingering developmental gaps.

Learning to Choose

All adults may not be capable of independent choices about living and working, though all should develop skills to their maximum capability. Most want to live independently, without parental influence or oversight. Life as an independent adult can be full of surprises, both exciting and frightening.

Parents need to overcome their fears about how much their retarded children can accomplish without them. This confidence is not always easily gained. Parents spend years being their children's advocate, protecting them from harm. Taking advantage of opportunities and services advancements means that parents must be ready to confront their own attitudes that may prevent or discourage their children from trying new options.

In the first half of the 20th century, most mentally retarded people resided at home or with relatives when parents died, or they lived in large institutions. The number of people with mental retardation living in institutions has declined markedly over the past 20 years, although this living option remains available in most states. Most professional organizations and consumer-directed advocacy groups do not view larger, congregate settings favorably. Conditions in mid-20th century institutions were often inhumane and abusive, reinforcing opposition to them.

With introduction of federal regulations in the 1970s, improvements in facility services emerged gradually. Enactment of the Civil Rights of Institutionalized Persons Act of 1980 (CRIPA) brought federal oversight into public institutions. Through the United States Department of Justice, Office of Civil Rights, the government broadened its ability to monitor and correct egregious civil rights violations. The home and community-based program, combined with numerous exposés on institutional abuses, accelerated states' efforts to expand housing options.

From 1960 on, new options emerged. Institutional placement, once the only out-of-home setting, became limited and is no longer provided by all states. Institutions have been replaced by varied public and private options: residences of small groups from two to six individuals; two or more people living as housemates; a home purchased by an individual or individuals; or supported living with specifically designed support services. With increased emphasis on self-determination, choice, and independence, options are now designed to support all ages and needs—from independence to 24-hour support needs.

The Fair Housing Act Amendments of 1988 prohibits public and private housing discrimination based on disability and other protected class designations such as color, familial status, race, religion, sex, or national origin. Further, housing discrimination is prohibited based on an individual's disability, that individual's association with a buyer or renter, or an individual with a disability who intends to live in the housing.

Home and Community-based Services

Beginning in 1981, the federal government authorized establishment of home and community-based services for people with disabilities. Today, programs throughout the United States serve over a quarter million Americans of many different ages and ability levels. Authorized as Medicaid-financed services, programs for those with mental retardation are provided in homes and communities rather than in long-term care facilities.

States are required to submit program plans for approval by the United States Department of Health and Human Services, Health Care Financing Administration (HCFA). Each state's plan and application procedures are different. Under Section 1915(c) of the Social Security Act, states may offer certain services such as adult day habilitation, case management, home health aid, personal care, and respite care. States must assure the federal government that the average cost of its home and community-based program will not exceed costs of state-provided institutional care. Parents should consult their state mental retardation authority or state protection and advocacy agency to learn more about their state plan options (see Appendix D).

Institutional Alternatives: the 1999 United States Supreme Court Decision

The development and provision of non-institutional services was the focus of a June 1999 ruling by the United States

Supreme Court that challenged states to prevent and correct inappropriate institutional placements. The Court's ruling also caused states to review intake and admissions procedures to ensure that people are offered living options with maximum community integration opportunities. States were obliged to provide places to live that are not isolated from other community residences.

In June 1999, the United States Supreme Court issued its ruling on Olmstead v. L.C. and E.W., a case brought by two Georgia women with mental retardation and mental illness who lived in a state institution. Facility team professionals determined that the women could live in a community residence. However, the state system placed the women on a community waiting list, lengthening their institutionalization by several years.

Assisted by Atlanta Legal Aid, the women sued, claiming that their continued involuntary residence violated their rights under the Americans with Disabilities Act of 1990 (ADA). The Court interpreted Title II of the ADA as the states' obligation to provide services, programs, and activities in the most integrated setting appropriate to the needs of qualified individuals with disabilities.

Under the Olmstead decision, states are now required to provide community-based services, using three guidelines for persons with disabilities: (1) professionals reasonably determine that the placement is appropriate, (2) the individual does not oppose the recommended service, and (3) the placement can be reasonably provided with due consideration for state resources and needs of other people who receive state-supported services.

The decision focused states on ensuring that decisions about where a person will live will be free of disability-based discrimination. Nationally, system changes sparked by this case are evolving. As no single state plan model was stipulated by the Court, states' responses have varied. For any qualified individual, particularly an adult who can live in the community, the ruling broadened both the expectation of and access to a place more homelike than an institution. However, the Court did not find that the ADA requires people to be moved from institutions when they are not able to manage or benefit from less restrictive living arrangements. Further, the Court did not imply service modifications beyond the fundamental capacity of a state's services, programs, or activities.

It's More Than Finding a House, It's a Way of Living

Choosing one's home and community without regard to disability is preferred by most citizens. Most people with mental retardation live either with their parents, siblings, or in their own homes. Choosing where to live is an individualized decision based on preferences, support needs, finances, location of work site, and community of residence. Because no single model or plan works for everyone, plans should be flexible. People may not like a selected option, have disagreements with housemates, or need more support than originally thought. In this regard, people and others who support housing choices must consider changes when the individual moves to the residence.

Questions need to be asked about the individual's leisure interests, available transportation, possible structural modifications for accessibility, how the individual will pay for rental, leasing or purchase, whether the individual wants or needs a housemate or live-in support staff, and location of other service supports. In lieu of independent housing, adults with mental retardation may live with their family and receive supports, such as day activities in a structured program.

Prior to a meeting to plan for future housing opportunities, people with retardation should be asked whom they want to invite, preferably people who know them well and who can provide information that will contribute to the plan's success. During the meeting, participants may realize that the individual has short-term needs that must be resolved before longer-term goals can be met. Considering the present living arrangement, participants may suggest interim options to acquire skills needed for more independent options.

Congregate housing settings

Housing options for people with mental retardation range from traditional institutions to smaller homes for four or more people. In these settings, staff provide 24-hour support, instruction in activities of daily living, and medical care. Again, proponents of total independence do not regard congregate settings as appropriate for people with mental retardation, even people with pervasive support needs.

Supported living settings

States provide a variety of housing programs for retarded individuals. In addition, the United States Housing and Urban Development Authority (HUD) provides grants to approved non-state organizations under the Section 811 Supportive Housing Options for Persons with Disabilities Program. Only eligible 501(c)(3) organizations may apply. Certain rental subsidies may also be available. Consumers may learn more about locally available HUD approved or subsidized housing by contacting their local or state HUD authority.

Supported options may include foster homes, apartments, or shared housing. A retarded individual may share a home with someone with a disability or with a live-in support person. People may live with a foster family who provides supervision and help in accessing community support. They may live in supported apartment settings with regular planned assistance. In states with approved voucher programs, those eligible may apply for funds to interview, hire, and pay salaried personal attendants who provide specific in-home support.

Independent living settings

During the past decade, people with mental retardation and their families sought alternatives to group homes. Today, they purchase or rent a neighborhood residence. In some communities with wider accessibility of apartments or condominiums, people may prefer ownership or rental without the added potential burdens of lawn care, home maintenance, or repair needs.

Home ownership brings added privacy, tremendous pleasure, and responsibilities—notably, understanding complex purchase and ownership details. Certainly, personal residence ownership offers greater control over life without interruptions, consideration of staff schedules, or other activities of group living settings. A carefully designed, active support system will be invaluable in helping the retarded individual reach an informed decision about such issues. The individual, the family, and support personnel must consider factors influencing housing decisions:

- The desirability of each living option
- Individual ability to establish and maintain a primary residence
- Possible barriers and resolution of barriers prior to seeking home ownership
- Behavioral, medical, or physical support needs
- Service system capabilities to meet support needs
- Needed funds for down payment or monthly mortgage payments

- Support network of sufficient strength to function for an indefinite period
- Provision for in-home supports
- Monitoring of financial means and needs
- Assistance with loan applications, tax and insurance documents, and related liability and legal issues

Competitive Employment

Competitive employment suggests that individuals have skills equivalent to those of workers without disabilities, a necessary attribute to be successful in today's workplace. Individuals with disabilities have specific workplace protections but are obliged to meet job requirements.

If a company has a history of affirmative hiring and accommodating work practices, its managers and supervisors tend to be more flexible than companies with little practical or positive experience in supporting mentally retarded workers. During the initial weeks on any job, both employees and their employers will benefit from an informally recognized get-acquainted period. Employees with mental retardation will need time to become part of the working group and accustomed to workplace routines, schedules, and procedures. Employers need to spend time getting to know the mentally retarded people they have hired, how those people work best, and what information they may need to fully understand their duties.

Supported Employment

The American Association on Mental Retardation defines "supported employment" as gainful competitive work in which supports assist a person in getting and keeping a job.

On-the-job support may mean that a job coach works with employees for an indefinite time to ensure that they are secure in performing assigned duties.

Unlike competitive employment, a job coach or other trained service provider will spend job time understanding the worker's specific goals. The job coach may demonstrate certain duties, provide verbal or physical guidance, provide suggestions to supervisors, and assess the worker's progress to greater independence.

Under the Rehabilitation Act Amendments of 1992, state vocational rehabilitation agencies may play a role in providing support. Individuals will be evaluated by those agencies to determine if they meets the requirements for receiving on-the-job assistance and other services. State vocational rehabilitation services must be provided as outlined in federal requirements. While a person may be eligible for on-the-job coaching or other support, assistance from state vocational rehabilitation agencies is a time-limited service.

Other Employment Options

Other employment options may provide more intensive daily support. In what is typically referred to as "sheltered workshops" or "work activity programs," workers may or may not have regular, salaried employment because these programs are dependent on area business and industry contracts. Professionals, advocacy organizations, and parents may not regard these work opportunities as bona fide employment because workers are isolated from the nondisabled in jobs that may not be the equivalent of true work. These objections are sometimes well-founded. "Practicing work" can hardly be regarded as a real job. Not all such programs devote adequate instruction and preparation to meaningful job-related skill development, job exploration, or activities to better acquaint workers with competitive and supported employment opportunities. Once in a segregated work program, many retarded adults have little or no means to move to other opportunities.

Parents and the mentally retarded worker must determine what services best meet strengths, needs, values, and life goals. Whatever the setting, services should contribute to that future vision. Work heightens personal satisfaction, self-worth, independence, and financial support. People with mental retardation should not be denied any resource that helps them further those aspirations.

Finding, Getting, and Keeping a Job

Mentally retarded people often find jobs through newspaper advertisements, family and friend referrals, or with assistance of teachers or other public agencies. Young adults with mental retardation often need assistance to make a successful transition to work. Helping such young people narrow the search is essential. They need to understand that they must be able to demonstrate that they are the most qualified individual for the job. While in transition activities, they should receive pre-employment skill instruction: locating potential jobs, developing a résumé, completing applications, preparing for and going to an interview, answering questions about career expectations, and marketing their skills.

Certain skills are expected of all workers. A desirable employee comes to work consistently and on time, works effectively and cooperatively, remains drug-free, follows supervisory instructions, and completes assigned work accurately. Unfortunately, not all young adults, including those with mental retardation, possess or understand the relative importance of these skills in finding and keeping their desired job.

Once hired, keeping a job means knowing and using the workplace skills that a particular employer values and federal and state laws require. In today's work environments, people are expected to work with those of different abilities, cultures, sexes, ages, and ethnic backgrounds. Federal employment laws have set certain conditions for public and private employment sites. These laws protect individuals in defined protected classes and prohibit derogatory or demeaning verbal and non-verbal behaviors toward co-workers, supervisors, and customers. Employers have a legal responsibility for enforcing federal and state laws in their workplace. Companies and organizations expect that workers will resolve disagreements or conflicts without yelling, hitting another person, or creating disruptions. Most companies have employee handbooks or policy guides that inform workers of their responsibilities to the employer, co-workers, and customers. Employees are expected to abide by applicable work laws and expectations that prohibit racial discrimination or sexual harassment in the workplace. Adults with disabilities are held to the same standard of behavior as other workers with regard to these legal requirements.

Enjoying Community Life

Being part of a community has different meanings for different people. For some individuals who enjoy the relative contentment of solitude, reading or gardening offers great personal satisfaction. Others find the companionship and conversation of friends to be energizing and stimulating. People who do not readily choose these activities, however, may feel frustrated and isolated from the kind of life that others enjoy.

Research suggests that adults with disabilities have fewer choices of activities. Their inability to participate in a community's social and recreational events may be due to a number of factors: lack of a supporting friendship network, lack of transportation, inadequate personal funds, inability to cultivate and maintain personal relationships, or lack of knowledge about how to find recreational activities. This may result in adults remaining dependent on family or paid care givers to support and share their recreational or leisure interests. On balance, depending on this network is not necessarily detrimental.

The lack of choices limits self-esteem. Faced with dependency on others, the mentally retarded may accept another person's choice rather than remain at home with few alternatives.

Access to and use of personal transportation may create nearly insurmountable challenges. In areas where public transportation is non-existent or minimal, dependency on other people may limit access to activities and events. Even with accessible public transportation, some adults are not skilled in using this community resource. Parents should insist that transition include using public transportation to get to work and community events either with or without family and friend support.

Developing friendships is an important avenue to greater leisure interests. Having a companion with whom one shares common interests makes recreational outings more enjoyable. How does a person with mental retardation learn to meet and make friends? How do they learn to interpret another person's behavior that tells them that their friendship is valued? Learning to find and maintain friends and read social cues is not always easy. These valuable skills must be acquired and honed over time.

It's a Big World: Staying Healthy, Staying Safe

Adults with mental retardation may overlook obvious dangers and become victims of robbery, assault, or other personal injury.

They may become targets of criminal activity simply because they tend to present little resistance or threat to an attacker. They may be threatened by a natural tendency to agree with other people without fully understanding what is being asked or said. In situations where there is risk of personal injury or physical threat, compliant attitudes and behaviors are maladaptive.

Film and television media have reinforced the idea that mentally retarded people are as gullible and unsuspecting as small children. For example, their testimony in legal matters is often overlooked or discounted because of their disability and its perceived effects on understanding the world around them.

Personal safety training needs to begin at an early age and need not be complicated or frightening. When living independently or with a house mate, adults need simple guidelines about how to control who comes into their homes, answering unknown callers at the door or on the telephone, and what to do if a person gets into their home without permission. This information should be provided in concrete, easy-to-remember terms.

Parents are well aware that young children must be taught to protect their bodies from uninvited abuse or attacks, to inform a trusted person of such advances, and to trust their instinct for self-protection. Adults with mental retardation may be vulnerable to greater insults simply because they may be easily influenced to allow their personal safety to be compromised. They should be taught that they do not have to become sexually intimate to be accepted, loved, or to have a relationship, and that immediate sexual access to their bodies can be a form of exploitation. Moreover, both young men and women should understand that sexual intercourse with someone whom they do not know well incurs the possibility of sexually transmitted or life-threatening diseases.

If a young person is sexually active, parents or guardians must assume an active role in sex education, including explaining the sexual act in concrete, anatomically correct terms, demonstrating and explaining how to use condoms, birth control pills, or other birth control methods. Young women need to learn essential facts about menstruation, reproduction, and family planning. Young men need to learn that they have an equal role in these topics.

Police and Fire Protection: What to Do In an Emergency

Emergency preparedness training has become greatly simplified with the advent of the 911 phone service. Knowing how and when to use 911 services is an important aspect of living in the community and should be taught to mentally retarded adults.

When looking for a potential home or apartment, determine the nearest police and fire stations. As a resource, local law enforcement and fire protection personnel can be helpful in teaching about a particular area, home safety and security, fire protection and prevention, and other information needed for personal safety.

Understanding the Law: Knowing Rights and Responsibilities

People with mental retardation possess the same rights and responsibilities as provided to other U.S. citizens by the United States Constitution. Mentally retarded adults are expected to obey laws that govern civil behavior and prohibit criminal activity.

State and federal laws regard everyone, including those with mental retardation, as competent until and unless certain conditions are demonstrated by the individual. A person may be found "incompetent" if the individual is adjudged unable to make independent decisions or future plans, shows very limited understanding of the results of personal behavior, and is deemed unable to choose, reason, and remember. Issues of individual competency must be proved in legal proceedings according to the laws of that state. Information about state competency laws and legal requirements may be obtained by contacting a state's bar association or legal aid association.

Guardianship: Determining the Need for an Appointed Caretaker

People with mental retardation capable of making independent decisions may need only infrequent assistance of family, friends, or advocacy organizations rather than a guardian. They may be able to make informed decisions about certain life needs and yet still need help to determine other decisions. For example, a person may understand and agree to a surgical procedure, but not understand the risks involved in surgery. They may understand that they earn a salary for work but not understand financial matters involved in purchasing a home.

Just as states' adjudication laws differ, guardianship laws differ. In most states, guardians must be appointed in a designated court proceeding that will detail personal matters that will fall under the guardian's oversight. Often, parents assume that their biological or family relationship provides the same authority and protections as a court-appointed guardian. In most states, a parent's relationship to an adult is just that—a parent, not with guaranteed legal authority to speak for and on behalf of their son or daughter. If parents are concerned about whether guardianship is warranted for their child, they should seek legal guidance about their state's requirements before their son or daughter reaches the age of majority.

Health Care: Uunderstanding Informed Consent for Medical Care

The advanced health care options and services available mean that people must be better informed and more assertive about health care provided by physicians and hospitals. Medical advances bring renewed concerns about informed consent issues. In light of the complex nature of American and state health care laws, individuals must be their own advocates when seeking medical opinions or treatment.

Counseling physicians should work with parents or family members prior to beginning medical care or treatment. Health care providers should consider specific questions:

- Is the person of majority age?
- Does the individual have enough relevant information about the proposed procedure?
- Is the person judged to be competent?
- Does the individual understand what has been shared about the medical care or treatment?
- Does the individual ask questions that demonstrate understanding of the medical care and its results?
- When provided information about any options, can the individual make reasoned decisions based on that information?
- Has the individual reached a decision without being forced or persuaded to choose a certain course of action?

If the person is judged not competent, alternatives may be sought that can support medical care decisions. Within states' laws, a legally appointed guardian may be empowered to make such decisions. Under those circumstances, guardians are responsible to make decisions in the best interests of the mentally retarded patient. When evaluating treatment options, guardians are obliged to consider the individual's recovery, pain, discomfort, risks, future health, and life expectancy with or without the treatment.

American society has become sensitized to the significance of advance directives and end-of-life treatment issues; many states have enacted laws that deal with those concerns. Providing clear written, authorized documents to health care providers and family members is vital should anyone become unable to voice preferences for medical treatment.

Capital Punishment

While states may differ in their interpretations and definition of "competence," state and federal laws ban certain acts. For people convicted and sentenced to death for capital crimes, imposition of the death penalty has generated much debate. Legal scholars point to the higher percentage of people with mental retardation in criminal justice and correctional systems. Advocacy organizations attribute the disparity to the willingness of retarded individuals to agree with someone in authority and follow that person's dictates without a clear understanding of the possible repercussions. These factors, and executions of people with mental retardation, have fueled loud opposition to and protests against the death penalty. Some states prohibit capital punishment of individuals with mental retardation convicted of crimes, and in June 2002, the U.S. Supreme court ruled that the execution of convicted felons with mental retardation violates the Constitution's ban on "cruel and unusual" punishment. The Court did not stipulate the criteria by which the determination of mental retardation would be made, although the language was reminiscent of that used in the AAMR definition. Opponents of the ruling fear that differences of opinion regarding what constitutes "mental retardation" and the potential for "malingering" during evaluations may produce a tangled web of endless court proceedings.

7. The Elderly

Before the 1950s, people with mental retardation usually died relatively young due to complications of multiple medical conditions that seem to cluster with mental retardation. In general, they represented one of the most vulnerable segments of the population.

More recently their life expectancy has expanded to very nearly that of the general population. Simultaneously, families began a search for more and different services. They lobbied for educational and vocational opportunities and pushed for living options to replace institutional care for all but the most severely disabled.

As longevity has increased in the general population, concern for the rights and quality of life of the elderly became an important issue. The same held true for those with mental retardation.

As baby boomers with mental retardation move from young adulthood to midlife, those who have mental retardation are caught in a time warp. They came along before special education was a mandate; educational opportunities were marginal, and their access to systematic vocational and occupational training was virtually nonexistent. As adults and children, they remained the responsibility of their families unless they were placed in one of the large state-run institutions for the mentally retarded.

Nevertheless, many individuals with limited support needs (i.e., the mildly retarded) achieved relative success in adjusting to adult life, living independently (or semi-independently), building personal and community relationships, and even sustaining employment and forming families of their own. Many managed independent or semi-independent lives of meaning, purpose, and satisfaction, not through the benevolence of government but through individual and family persistence. Strengthened by close-knit, supportive families and communities (especially rural communities), people were accepted as productive, employed community members.

Nevertheless, as a group, baby boomers with retardation are more likely to have been maintained in dependent family or institutional circumstances than to be educated and provided vocational training. As a result, many now face difficult transitions to midlife as family caretakers suffer ill health and are no longer able to care of them.

Boomers who have been institutionalized over long periods generally have been conditioned to survive, and perhaps to thrive, in those settings. Those same skills do not serve them as well as successive new waves of self-determination, vocational and occupational training, and community adjustment ideologies move through the system. For these boomers, the types of institutional and community services now available at times seem too little, too late.

What Do Older Adults Need to Build and Maintain a Fulfilling Life?

As Stanley S. Herr and Germain Weber noted eloquently in their 1999 text *Aging, Rights, and Quality of Life*, "It takes more than compassion to let hidden people bloom."

People have similar basic needs regardless of their mental capacity. In the United States, federal and state mandates essentially ensure that individuals with mental retardation have sufficient financial resources to meet their basic needs for food, water, and clothing. Housing, safety, health care, and social needs are met through a variety of means.

Housing and Safety

The mentally retarded aging face changes in housing needs earlier than the general population, often in midlife. Three factors tend to force abrupt decisions regarding living arrangements: severe illness or death of caretaker parent(s), development of severe physical health problems, and onset of significant cognitive and/or behavioral symptoms.

Reared by protective (perhaps overprotective) parents, these adults seem unprepared for life. Individuals who were over-protected often developed a "functional" retardation in addition to their intrinsic mental disability. They may be unable to take initiative and to care for themselves. They may not learn how to judge dangers and protect themselves, and instead wait to be told when, where, and how to do things. They often come to fear decision making because they have little experience with it.

Through a lifetime of focused care by their parents, these middle-aged adults have become accustomed to constant attention and supervision. When that ends, middle-aged adults may find themselves moved to institutional settings where they may become semi-anonymous members of a group (sometimes a large group), no longer the center of attention and supervised. Such changes are often emotionally traumatic and can be catastrophic.

Parents often expect that siblings eventually will assume care for the retarded adult. Usually these expectations are not communicated and not formalized. When siblings do take on responsibility, they usually procure or manage care rather than assume it directly.

Much happier are the situations in which parents provided instruction along with protection, emancipation along with nurturing. Some adults were fortunate enough to be enrolled in appropriate educational programs by parents who turned their own persistence and creativity toward finding vocational and occupational training for their child. Those adults were challenged to expand their range and to learn skills needed for community living, maximizing their capabilities to move into more independent or semi-independent living arrangements.

Living arrangements vary according to individual abilities. People encouraged to reach their full potential may live in a variety of settings with varying degrees of independence and supervision: community group homes, supervised apartments, homes of extended family or friends, or single-family housing with minimum assistance by family and community.

Many people with mild mental retardation (such as those with Down syndrome) can live relatively independently in private or public housing with some community-based services provided to assist them; they manage their own budgets, pay their own bills, prepare meals, do their own laundry and household chores, and even hold part- or full-time jobs and pay taxes, all with only occasional and unintrusive assistance from others.

Individuals with moderate mental retardation (such as those with fragile X syndrome or Prader-Willi syndrome), and to some extent those with severe mental retardation, can live in supervised group home arrangements, enjoying the benefits of more privacy and a community environment.

Individuals acculturated to independent or semi-independent living are not as vulnerable to emotional trauma when their living arrangements are changed. They are less likely to find themselves in institutional environments upon the illness or deaths of their parents.

Adults with moderate retardation who have significant behavior problems or those with profound retardation (who usually have multiple, significant medical problems) may continue to live in structured settings where more intensive levels of medical and psychiatric/psychological intervention, occupational and recreational therapy are available on a consistent basis.

Health Care

As will be discussed more thoroughly in chapter 8, individuals with mental retardation tend to be at greater risk for developing additional brain dysfunction that tends to cause significant behavior changes. The frequency of various mental illnesses and Alzheimer dementia are increased in the population with mental retardation. This group also tends to exhibit cognitive and behavioral deterioration at an earlier age. Individuals with Down syndrome may experience a decrease in daily living skills, functional abilities, and an onset of behavior problems in their early thirties. They also have a greater risk for developing Alzheimer dementia and tend to develop the symptoms earlier than their counterparts in the general population.

In general, the more severe the mental retardation, the more likely individuals are to have multiple, significant medical and dental problems, but people with retardation tend to be more intimidated by doctors and nurses. Perhaps because of their anxiety, they may be less able to explain their physical symptoms. They may answer "yes" to every question posed by the health care staff or refuse to speak at all, causing confusion and frustration that may further complicate their diagnosis and treatment.

As the aging process progresses, symptoms may go unreported in individuals with limited communication skills.

Caretakers should tell health care personnel to be alert to changes in the patient's facial expressions and behavior that may signify physical discomfort.

One area of treatment that appears to be different for those with mental retardation is dementia. Current therapies do not seem to meet the needs of individuals with mental retardation who develop symptoms of dementia. Medications that postpone (but not cure) the rapid advancement of Alzheimer dementia usually are not given to those with retardation and advancing memory problems.

The greater risk of physical and intellectual decline for the mentally retarded in midlife forces consideration of more supervised care, in residential facilities or community group homes designed specifically for those with mental retardation or in nursing home facilities.

As aging proceeds, cognitive decline may progress to the point where inborn capacity and education are no longer relevant. Advanced Alzheimer dementia symptoms are the same with and without mental retardation. Patients are confused and their behaviors are unpredictable and disordered. At that point, the primary problem becomes the dementia rather than their previous state.

Clinical experience indicates that, as their mental and physical health decline, many of the mentally retarded are not deemed eligible or suitable for nursing home placement. In many cases, clinicians suspect that the diagnosis of mental retardation is the stumbling block, rather than the current status of the individual. In other words, old stigmas re-emerge even in the determination of who will receive medical care in an extended nursing facility during the twilight years of life. Application of the Olmstead decision, discussed in chapter 6, may level the playing field.

Social Integration

Humans are a gregarious species and people with mental retardation are no exception. Older people are particularly vulnerable to social isolation. Yet somehow, in designing supports, service providers (and occasionally even families) sometimes underestimate the need for companionship. In their text *Community Supports for Aging Adults with Lifelong Disabilities* (2000), Matthew P. Janicki and Edward F. Ansello note that perspectives of older adults and their service providers often differ with regard to social integration. Janicki and Ansello report that service providers tend to focus more on residential settings (i.e., group homes, parents' homes) and the community (i.e., rural communities more than urban communities) while older adults with mental retardation focus more on their places of work than on their residential settings as the most common venues for making friends and blending socially. In fact, many individuals working in "sheltered workshops" for those with mental retardation complain of boredom, but continue to go to work because of the daily opportunities to socialize.

Recreation is another area where service providers and their clients hold different views. Janicki and Ansello concluded that older adults with mental retardation tend to view solitary activities at home as recreational, an outlet that providers often overlook. While both recognize recreation as a facilitator of social integration, providers tend to discuss the issue in general terms while their clients focus on the importance of having structured recreational opportunities as well as solitary activities at home.

Another contrasting perspective is the way friends are defined. Older people with mental retardation tend to consider their service providers as friends, while the service providers believe that relationships with paid staffers are not "true" friendships. They believe that these singular relationships do not enhance social integration. Nevertheless, the friendship value of service providers to clients should not be underestimated.

Retirement

Retirement is often postponed for people with mental retardation enrolled in work opportunity programs. Apparently, service providers unconsciously overlook the age of clients with whom they have worked with for years. Thus, the behavior specialist continues to include employment in the person-centered planning as the years pass, forgetting that people 65 years or greater generally prefer to retire.

Person-centered planning should reflect the changing life stage of elder adults. Instead of work, opportunities for structured recreation should be bolstered in order to maintain the social skills of retirement-aged clients who no longer wish to be employed on a daily basis.

Planning by Parents

According to A. Richardson and J. Ritchie (1986; 1989), parents maintain one of three attitudes toward planning for the future of their children when they themselves can no longer provide direct care: avoidance, ambivalence, or active planning—avoidance being the most common. They noted that only one third to one half of parents make concrete plans for future care of their children with mental retardation. Financial planning is the most common type of planning undertaken.

When plans are made, the alternatives often are not discussed with the adult child. Frequently, families disregard the preferences of their child if these are incompatible with the attitudes of the parents.

Richardson and Ritchie also reported that parental preferences for future care of adult children with mental retardation are generally evenly split between continued family care (primarily by siblings) and residential placement. Findings consistently showed that, although elderly parents often do attempt to make plans for later care of their adult children, they prefer to provide direct care themselves so long as they are physically able.

Richardson and Ritchie also found that parents value protection and permanency in placement opportunities for their adult children over developmental opportunities. They perceive that their adult children gradually will become more dependent as they age. The parents therefore seek future residential placement opportunities that would duplicate the care they have given in their own homes.

Dealing with Grief

People with mental retardation experience the same stages of grief as do people in the general population. According to most authorities, the major difference is the fact that those with more pervasive disability rely on nonverbal communication to express their emotional upheaval. Some differences may exist in grief expression based on the differences in life experiences and culture. In this context, culture must include whether individuals were reared within families or in institutions.

Frequently, when family members die, adults with mental retardation are not invited to join in the socially sanctioned rites of mourning. They are told of the death after the fact, often with the stated intent of protecting them. Another underlying motivation of distraught family members may simply be that they do not want to take on additional stressful responsibility for one whose reactions may be unpredictable or disturbing.

Optimally, such life events provide role models for grieving and emotionally healthy opportunities for the family member with mental retardation to vent grief in a socially, emotionally acceptable fashion. Janicki and Ansello suggest the following measures that care providers can take to assist retarded individuals who are grieving:

- Develop nonverbal, symbolic rituals for grieving, particularly for those individuals who cannot participate in or find no comfort in verbal rituals,
- Respect both the avoidance of photos and memorabilia as well as the choice of same,
- Minimize major changes in the individual's environment and program for at least a year,
- Postpone assessment of skills and behaviors,
- Assist appropriate searching behavior to support emotional recovery,
- Support formal observation of birthdays and other significant anniversaries associated with the memory of the deceased, and
- Seek consultation with specialists in grief counseling if behavior changes occur, such as mutism, aggression, depression, regression, self-injury, wandering, and tearfulness.

These authors note that an individual's developmental stage determines the manner of their grieving, not whether or not grief is felt. Will such a sad event be overly stimulating for someone with immature impulse control? Will the event be an opportunity for family to come together? The intellectual level of an individual does determine to a significant degree the extent of the individual's understanding of death. Still, except for those with pervasive support needs, the signs of grief are universal: tears, sorrow, anger, disbelief, and panic.

When death of a loved one is anticipated, advance counseling may help prepare an individual for coming loss and grief. Certainly, open discussion will help diminish the overwhelming shock component.

When possible, people with mental retardation should be allowed to participate in the grieving process, including the social rites. Service providers, clergy, and families can help them deal with the grief process and provide support during the formal death ceremonies.

8. Psychiatric Illness and Mental Retardation

Mental retardation is associated with an increased risk for other disorders that originate in the brain, including seizure disorders and mental or behavioral disorders. The term "dual diagnosis" is now frequently used to refer to the simultaneous presence of mental illness with another serious disorder, such as mental retardation.

Mental illnesses are severe disturbances in mood, behavior, and/or thought processes that usually result in significant social and interpersonal difficulties. Most of the mental illnesses that afflict the general population also occur in people with mental retardation, often with increased frequency.

Prior to the 1970s, clinicians working with retarded individuals tended to explain the behavioral or mental problems they experienced as symptoms of their mental retardation. The more bizarre symptoms were diagnosed as psychosis due to mental retardation. Because mood disorders were diagnosed rarely in this group, mood symptoms were either ignored or suppressed by the use of restrictive environmental measures, sedating tranquilizers, or both.

In the 1970s, clinicians began to recognize that mental illness can occur in association with mild mental retardation. Given the relatively good communication skills of people with mild retardation, clinicians found they could apply criteria for diagnosis of mental disorders to both the general population and to those with mild forms of retardation. The use of treatment modalities found effective in adults and children without intellectual deficits (including more discriminating use of medications) proved beneficial in individuals with mental retardation who exhibited clear symptoms of mental illness.

It has only been within the past fifteen years that clinicians have attempted more precise diagnostic assessment of people with moderate to severe mental retardation who have symptoms not entirely explained by their developmental deficits. One major difficulty in making accurate psychiatric diagnoses in individuals with moderate and more severe mental retardation is their limited language skills.

Diagnostic Criteria for Mental Illness

The two commonly used classification systems for diagnosis of mental disorders in the U.S. are the Diagnostic and Statistical Manual of Mental Disorders, Fourth Edition (DSM-IV-TR) and the International Classification of Diseases, Tenth Edition (as discussed in chapter 3). The criteria of both systems rely heavily on the presence of intact language skills, a circumstance that produces obvious difficulties for clinicians attempting to diagnose people with moderate to profound mental retardation who have limited or absent language skills. For example, a clinician assessing an adult with no intellectual deficits may note unusually rapid speech ("pressured" speech) that is rambling and long-winded ("flight of ideas") and contains unusual elements of grossly inflated self-worth (grandiose delusions) or illogical ideas of persecution (paranoid delusions). These observations of abnormalities in form, flow, and content of speech patterns coincide with required criteria for the diagnosis of bipolar disorder, according to DSM-IV. When hyperactivity is also present, the clinician may suspect that the individual is suffering from mania, one of the abnormal mood states of bipolar disorder.

Suppose the clinician assesses a hyperactive adult with moderate to severe mental retardation and very limited (or no) language skills. How can pressured speech or flight of ideas be noted? It is impossible to judge the rationality of speech that does not exist. The clinician is thus left attempting to interpret behavior that is overactive, disorganized, impulsive, destructive, or aggressive relative to the individual's usual baseline behavior. Often, the clinician will find it difficult to judge where the individual's baseline level of function lies unless someone familiar with the person being assessed is available to describe the "usual" behavior versus the "new" behavior. Interpretations aside, the clinician still will not be able to apply the primary criteria for bipolar illness because these require the presence of symptoms that are based on what individuals say and the way they say it.

Mental health clinicians now attempt to differentiate between the intellectual and behavioral functions of individuals with mental retardation and the changes in brain function and behavior associated with mental illness. It is necessary to use standard diagnostic criteria, as poorly suited as they may be to people with mental retardation. Approximation is the key.

Impact of Mental Retardation on Presentation of Psychiatric Symptoms

Mental retardation can obscure the presenting symptoms of mental illness. R. Sovner identified four characteristics of mental retardation that contribute to difficulties in the diagnosis of coexisting psychiatric conditions:

Intellectual distortion
Individuals with mental retardation experience difficulties describing emotional symptoms because of limitations in abstract thinking and in both receptive and expressive language

skills. People with more severe forms of mental retardation do not verbalize complaints of anxiety or depression.

Psychosocial masking

The limited social experiences of many individuals with retardation often influence the content of psychiatric symptoms. For example, people with moderate mental retardation coexisting with psychotic disorders rarely report being monitored by the CIA or the FBI, a common complaint of paranoid members of the general population. Instead, they may express the delusional belief that someone is "messing" with them or stealing from them.

Cognitive disintegration

A common attribute of mental retardation is a decreased ability to tolerate stress. Under stress, people with mental retardation may experience anxiety leading to disorganization in their thinking and behavior that can be misinterpreted as psychosis.

Baseline exaggeration

Many individuals with retardation exhibit a long-term pattern of maladaptive behavior. If they develop a psychiatric disorder, the primary change in their condition may be an increase in severity or frequency of the previously existing maladaptive symptoms.

Mental Retardation and Mental Illness

Some authorities believe the rate of psychiatric disorders in individuals with mental retardation may be four to five times greater than that in the general population. An estimated

10–40% of individuals with mental retardation have diagnosable mental illnesses (Reiss, 1990).

The symptoms of emotional disorders in people with mild mental retardation are indistinguishable from those seen in mentally ill people of normal intelligence. The same may not be true of psychiatric disorders occurring in people with more profound intellectual deficits. In these, symptoms of mental illness may manifest as behavioral changes or exaggerations of previously existing behaviors. Sometimes these changes occur precipitously and therefore may be quickly recognized and addressed. Often, however, the changes caused by mental illness may be subtle at the outset and progress slowly, so that factors other than mental illness may be blamed.

Most people with mental retardation and psychiatric illness can be managed as outpatients in their community although some may require temporary residential or hospital care. Nonmedication interventions may help reduce the impact of environmental stresses that can precipitate or aggravate mental illness. Expert, multidisciplinary community teams involved in the habilitation of individuals with mental retardation provide the best opportunity for maximizing abilities and enhancing quality of life in a community environment. These teams are usually supplemented by mental health professionals, such as psychologists and psychiatrists, when mental illness is also a factor. Medical specialists, such as neurologists, may also be on the team.

People with mental retardation who suffer from chronic, severe mental illnesses (mood disorders, psychoses, and violent or self-abusive behavior) may benefit from the day-to-day services of behavioral specialists provided in residential or psychiatric inpatient facilities. This is especially true when difficulties have occurred or are anticipated with medication stabilization. Safety issues are often the ultimate reasons for treatment in a controlled environment provided by a residential or psychiatric inpatient facility.

Psychoeducational Intervention

As a result of federal legislation, children and adolescents with mental retardation or related developmental disorders (including mental illness) are entitled to free intervention based on their needs as determined by a team of professionals. Such interventions should address the priorities and concerns of the family and be provided in the least restrictive and most inclusive setting (i.e., where the children have every opportunity to benefit from interacting with nondisabled peers and the community resources available to all children).

Infant and toddler services

Services to infants and toddlers can be home-based, center-based, or some combination of the two. The nature of the services should be based on results of the child's assessment and family priorities for the child. The results, in turn, will be used to develop an Individual Family Service Plan for the child, as described in chapter 4.

Preschool and school services

Services to preschool children, ages 3 years through 5 years, and school-age children, 6 through 21 years, can be home-based, but are more frequently center-based. The Individualized Education Plan (IEP), described in chapter 3, details the objectives for improving the child's skills and may include family- or parent-focused activities. Services should be provided in the most inclusive, least restrictive setting, such as a regular preschool program, Head Start center, or the child's home.

Social/interpersonal intervention

Group social and recreational activities can be both preventative and therapeutic and should be a component of the child's educational program. These activities should include nondisabled peers and may include participation in recreational activities such as birthday parties, youth sports, movies, and community-sites visits such as the zoo. The goal should be to teach appropriate social skills relevant to group participation and building self-esteem.

Parents may benefit from prevention activities. Respite care provided by trained individuals can afford parents the opportunity to address their own needs (e.g., personal time, medical appointments, socializing with peers, etc.). Social or parent support groups can also be an outlet for parents to discuss their feelings with others who have similar experiences.

Child behavioral interventions can be used to teach self-care, vocational, leisure, interpersonal, and survival skills (e.g., finding a public restroom). Disruptive behaviors such as tantrums, self-injury, noncompliance, and aggression can also be addressed through behavioral techniques. The most frequent form of behavioral intervention for problematic behavior involves differential reinforcement of problem behaviors (Batshaw & Perret, 1992).

Assessment of coexisting psychiatric disorders and mental retardation

Appropriate assessment of psychiatric disorders in people with dual diagnosis is important because accurate assessment can suggest the form of treatment, may ensure access to and funding for special services, and can be used to evaluate subsequent interventions (Sturmey, 1995).

Brain damage, epilepsy, and language disorders are risk factors for psychiatric disorders and are often associated with mental retardation (Rutter et al., 1976; Sturmey, 1995). Social isolation, stigmatization, and poor social skills put individuals with mental retardation at further risk for mood disorders (Reiss & Benson, 1985).

Children with mental retardation are diagnosed with psychiatric disorders more often than children without retardation. Both groups are usually diagnosed with the same types of disorders, except in the case of children with severe and profound levels of retardation where a tendency to uncommon psychiatric disorders exists (Batshaw & Perret, 1992). Often, these result in behaviors that are self-injurious: head-banging (sometimes to the point of mutilating the ears), rectal digging, self-biting (especially involving lips), and other self-mutilation.

Most psychologists and psychiatrists have little exposure to individuals with mental retardation and are sometimes uncomfortable treating them; in fact, many professionals seem unaware that these individuals can experience mental health problems (Reiss & Szyszko, 1983). Mental health and mental retardation systems have been separated in this country for many years, making it administratively difficult to serve people with both mental retardation and mental health disorders (Matson & Sevin, 1994). Recently, there has been heightened awareness of the need to pursue behavioral-psychiatric assessment, diagnosis, and treatment of people with retardation and mental health problems (Bregman, 1991; Eaton & Menolascino, 1982; Reiss, 1990).

Interdisciplinary approach

People with dual diagnosis are best served by an interdisciplinary team of specialists who, together with the individuals' families, provide assessment, planning, and implementation of habilitation plans to address both the developmental and the psychiatric aspects of the dual diagnosis. Behavioral analysis, psychoeducational assessment, speech and language testing, and medical and neurological assessments are also key components.

Psychiatric assessment

Psychiatric assessment can be stressful and performance levels are often below expectations due to anxiety. The manner in which a psychiatric assessment is performed is critical to obtaining an accurate idea of the symptoms experienced by anyone, especially an individual with mental retardation.

Assessment should occur in a safe, private, quiet setting that is neither distracting nor overstimulating. Some individuals deliberately "act out" (or "show out") to get attention when they have an audience; others become withdrawn and mute when flurries of unfamiliar people mill around. When possible, a member of the individual's family or a familiar staff person (or both) should remain and provide essential historical information. Attempts should be made to reassure all concerned.

Ideally, the individual, family, and staff should be seen promptly to avoid behavioral problems that may occur with boredom, increasing anxiety, or increasing frustration on the part of any of the three groups. The procedures involved in the assessment should be explained simply and carefully (as much as is practical) directly to the individual who is to be assessed. It is important to note that the receptive language skills of people with mental retardation may exceed their expressive language skills; they may understand far more than they can communicate.

Physical assessment is important in determining whether developing behavioral symptoms are caused by underlying medical problems or medication side effects. Physical conditions such as intermittent, severe constipation can cause such discomfort that nonverbal individuals may resort to aggression or self-injurious behaviors (SIBs) to deal with the frustration of unrelieved pain. Extreme restlessness accompanied by hand tremors, stepping in place, constant movements of extremities, and increased muscle tone may indicate the presence of side effects of antipsychotic medications that have been used to target "agitation." Lack of recognition that medication side effects may masquerade as agitation can result in a vicious cycle of increased medication followed by increased agitation followed by increased medication. Unrecognized or uncontrolled seizure activity can adversely affect mood, memory, and behavior.

Assessment should done in brief segments (30–60 minutes maximum) to limit performance deterioration. Care should be taken to double-check information because people with mental retardation tend to "endorse" all statements or symptoms. The assessment includes information about daily living skills (and recent changes), medications, medical history, developmental history, educational level, social skills, family history, and previous psychiatric assessments and treatment. Routine laboratory tests screen for medical illnesses (such as thyroid disease or vitamin B-12 deficiency) and environmental toxins (such as lead or mercury) that can cause mental retardation and psychiatric illness.

Psychiatric Disorders and Mental Retardation

Psychiatric disorders can be acute, chronic, or episodic. They can be due to environmental stresses or medical or physiological factors or a combination of both.

Anxiety disorders and mental retardation
Anxiety can be intermittent and situational or constant with periodic worsening, but never entirely absent, and can last for

weeks, months, or years. Some individuals complain of frequent physical ailments (e.g., headaches, stomachaches, dizziness, etc.) accompanied by varying degrees of nervousness. Still others experience abrupt, rapidly escalating bursts of fear associated with tingling around the mouth and in the fingers, light-headedness, difficulty breathing (often with hyperventilation), heart palpitations, and a sense of impending doom.

Anxiety experienced by individuals with moderate to severe retardation tends to be closely tied to environmental issues, but can be free-floating (i.e., without clear cause). Most commonly, it is evidenced by restless, tearful, avoidant, and occasionally aggressive or self-abusive behaviors that occur in response to anxiety-provoking situations. The more frightening the situation, the less effective the individual's normal defense mechanisms. The more limited the individual's intellectual capacity, the more likely that extreme behaviors will occur in response to noxious environmental stresses.

The key questions when individuals with moderate to profound retardation develop intermittent restlessness, tearfulness, and/or avoidant behaviors are pragmatic. Have there been any changes in the individual's environment? Medication changes? Changes in physical health? New people? Absence of trusted caretakers? Any question of victimization?

Obsessive compulsive disorder (or "OCD") is a subtype of anxiety disorder. It presents with a variety of repetitive, pervasive, usually disturbing thoughts (often involving shame or anxiety/fear) that roll over in the individual's mind like a broken record and cannot easily be banished. Commonly, individuals with obsessional thoughts also are plagued by repetitive (compulsive) behaviors that are not entirely within their control because significant anxiety results when attempts are made to suppress the compulsions. The presence of compulsions with no obsessional symptoms is rare.

Obsessions tend to fall into several broad categories: fear of germs or dirt or contamination, repeated doubts (especially self-doubts), need for symmetry and order, aggressive or violent images, or sexual images.

Compulsive behaviors are behavioral equivalents to obsessions. For instance, individuals with fears of contamination by dirt or germs may spend excessive amounts of time engaged in extensive, prolonged cleaning rituals, such as hand washing, or in avoiding potential contamination, such as by avoiding public restrooms. Similarly, people who experience obsessional self-doubting and obsessional fears of harm to self or others may engage in extensive checking/rechecking behaviors to reassure themselves (such as checking home appliances repeatedly to ensure that they are turned off). Other examples of compulsive behaviors include ritual bathing, repetitive spitting, repeated touching, insistence on sameness or symmetry, and compulsive collecting or hoarding of items (often with little value).

Some compulsions are primarily mental in nature. Individuals may silently repeat specific words (sometimes, "holy" words or prayers) or engage in compulsive spelling (or mental "typing") of words or compulsive mental arithmetic (such as adding the digits of automobile license tags or juggling phone number digits or columns of numbers until a "magic" number or sequence of numbers occurs).

OCD appears to be anxiety-driven; that is, increasing anxiety seems to make the symptoms worse. Likewise, attempts to suppress the symptoms tend to bring on increased anxiety. The disorder tends to wax and wane over time, even without treatment, and is associated with varying degrees of depression.

OCD versus stereotypy versus tics
Individuals with mental retardation often exhibit so-called "stereotypic" behaviors. Stereotypies are repetitive motor

behaviors that markedly interfere with normal activities or result in self-inflicted bodily injury. Stereotypic behaviors often have a compulsive quality and may include skin picking that produces lesions, hair pulling leaving bald areas on the scalp (referred to as trichotillomania), head banging, hand waving, rocking, playing with hands, fiddling with fingers, twirling objects, self-biting, hitting self (especially on the chest or head), eye gouging, and inserting foreign objects into body orifices (nose, mouth, ears, urethra, vagina, rectum). When the repetitive behaviors are severe enough to interfere with normal functioning or cause (or potentially cause) injury, the behaviors often become the focus of treatment. In general, the more severe the mental retardation, the greater the likelihood of self-injurious behaviors (SIBs). SIBs occur in individuals of all ages. Head banging is three times more common in males than in females, possibly because some of the severe disorders that result in head banging occur primarily in males (e.g., fragile X syndrome).

The difference between compulsions and stereotypies is a fine point that may be more semantic than real. Both result from abnormal brain functioning, although the exact nature and site of the brain malfunction has not yet been identified. In general, compulsions are more complex and ritualistic than stereotypies and are performed in response to an obsession or according to strictly applied rules.

Individuals occasionally demonstrate patterns of repetitive behaviors, such as touching or tapping portions of the body or pieces of clothing in a systematic, sequential manner repeatedly. These behaviors may preoccupy affected individuals and tend to disengage them from their environment.

Tics are neither stereotypies nor compulsions but are involuntary, repetitive muscle movements that often present with fatigue (e.g., tics of eyelids with eye strain) or are associated with identifiable neurological conditions. They may also be seen in highly anxious people who have no diagnosable neurological conditions.

Some individuals with mental retardation and stereotypies demonstrate self-restraining behaviors, presumably in an attempt to prevent self-injury. They may be seen to sit on their hands or to place their hands in pockets or shirts. In such cases, when self-restraint is prevented, problematic behaviors (such as SIBs) may recur.

Behavior programs can be effective at diminishing the frequency of (or entirely eliminating) compulsive and/or stereotypic behaviors. Behavior programs preferably should provide reinforcement for positive alternative behaviors rather than aversive responses to problem behaviors. Occasionally, when a repetitive behavior is eliminated by self-restraint or by behavior modification, another problem behavior develops in its place and becomes repetitive.

Mood disorders and mental retardation

Mood disorders occur commonly with mental retardation and involve disturbances in mood, thought processes, energy level, activity level, pleasure capacity, appetite, sleep, and sex drive. Feelings of helplessness, hopelessness, and worthlessness are common.

Behaviors that may represent "depressive equivalents" differ from the individual's baseline function and include sluggishness, decreased interest in previous activities, social isolation, weight loss, deterioration in performance of activities of daily living, sleep abnormalities (insomnia, interrupted sleep, excessive sleep), self-injurious behavior, and aggression.

When severely depressed, retarded individuals may hallucinate (usually hearing and seeing things that are not present). They may also become paranoid, believing things that are patently unlikely or untrue.

Depression may be mild, moderate, or severe; situational or "endogenous" (i.e., related primarily to biological factors); can occur as a single episode or as multiple episodes; and can be chronic and static or wax and wane but never completely disappear.

Bipolar disorder is a form of mood disorder that involves "mood swings," both "highs" (i.e., manic episodes) and "lows" (i.e., depressive episodes). Individuals with bipolar disorder experience episodes of depression as well as mania (i.e., periodic bursts of hyperactivity, irritability, elation, difficulty focusing on tasks, and marked decrease in the need for sleep). Mania can be mild (periods of enhanced self-esteem and increased energy and productivity coupled with a very limited need for sleep) or severe (unrealistically enhanced self-esteem, irritability and agitation with aggressive or destructive behavior, pressured speech, racing thoughts, hyperactivity, poor insight, decreasing ability to concentrate and to complete tasks, loss of need for sleep for several days, and poor judgment socially, sexually, and/or financially). Grandiose and/or paranoid delusions often occur with more severe mood swings and are sometimes accompanied by hallucinations, usually auditory.

Depression and bipolar disorder are common in people with mental retardation, but are often unrecognized in those with moderate to severe retardation. The risk for bipolar disorder in those with retardation is between 3% and 8%, significantly higher than for the general population where the risk is approximately one percent.

Periodic escalations of bizarre, hyperactive, irritable, intrusive, aggressive, or giggly behavior may be found to occur regularly on a seasonal basis if caregivers plot behavioral parameters along a time-line over a number of years. Clinical experience indicates that such episodes of probable undiagnosed mood swings tend to occur in spring or late summer.

Adjustment disorders and mental retardation

An acute adjustment disorder is an excessive emotional reaction to one or more stresses and, by definition, resolves within six months following relief from the stress. Occasionally, an adjustment disorder becomes chronic. Adjustment disorders are subtyped by their predominant symptoms; i.e., depressed mood, anxiety, mixed anxiety and depression, disturbance of conduct (a pattern of behavior problems that involves violation of the rights of others or violations of rule and accepted norms of society), or mixed disturbance of emotions and conduct.

Adjustment disorders commonly can be managed by supportive therapy and/or by environmental manipulation. When these methods do not alleviate adjustment disorder symptoms that significantly impair function, consideration should be given to time-limited use of medication to target the most troubling symptoms.

Psychotic disorders and mental retardation

Psychotic disorders (also called "psychoses") are severe forms of mental illness in which contact with reality is lost or severely impaired. Psychoses are characterized by delusions (e.g., false beliefs, not shared by the individual's culture, that cannot be dispelled by logic), hallucinations (perceptions that occur with no apparent stimulus, such as "voices" of people not present or "visions" of things or people not present), marked changes in mood, poor impulse control, behavior or remarks that seem "strange," and often disorganization of thought patterns. Psychoses are also usually associated with marked deterioration in behavior from a previously stable level of function.

Psychoses due to medical problems typically present with "delirium"—confusion manifested by short-term memory impairment, disorientation (to time and place and sometimes also to person and situation), as well as auditory and visual hallucinations. Individuals who have suffered prior insults to the brain (i.e., people with dementia, traumatic brain damage, or mental retardation) are more sensitive to those factors that may cause "organic" psychosis. When such symptoms appear, a thorough medical and laboratory assessment is warranted. In fact, when any individual presents with visual hallucinations in the absence of (or significantly more prominent than) auditory hallucinations, a medical cause for the psychosis should be sought.

Schizophrenia is a well-known form of psychosis the cause of which remains unknown. Schizophrenia is characterized by fundamental and often quite severe distortions of thinking and perception and by mood changes that are not appropriate to the social context (often flat and unchanging). Thoughts tend to be disorganized, illogical, and eccentric. As a result, affected individuals tend to perceive that others are reading or controlling or otherwise manipulating their thoughts; tend to give special, highly personal interpretations to mundane events (e.g., receiving special messages from the TV); and tend to produce loosely organized, difficult to follow, peculiar patterns of speech ("looseness of association").

Approximately 1% of people will develop schizophrenia over their lifetime. Among people with mental retardation, studies suggest that between 2% and 6% will develop schizophrenia. The diagnosis of schizophrenia is usually made only in symptomatic individuals with mild to moderate mental retardation.

Some experts in the field of mental retardation and developmental disabilities suggest that social and psychological factors (such as disadvantage, the effects of low self-esteem, stigma, and lack of empowerment) may play a role in the increased risk for psychosis in people with mental retardation. The greatest contributing factor, however, appears to be the presence of a disorder affecting the brain (such as epilepsy).

Presumably, the increased risk for schizophrenia and other psychoses in the population of individuals with mental retardation is caused by the inherent vulnerability of a brain already damaged, often by unknown factors.

The diagnosis of psychoses in individuals with mild retardation is usually not difficult for behavioral clinicians. The diagnosis can be more difficult in persons with more severe forms of retardation where language skills are likely to be limited. A change in mental functioning (such as the development of unusual preoccupations or fears) may be a clue to the development of psychosis, but care must be taken to differentiate the symptoms of psychosis from symptoms seen with other psychiatric disorders.

The treatment of psychoses is threefold:

• Protection of the individual and others from the impulsive behaviors rooted in irrational and/or fearful thoughts,
• Treatment of any underlying physical disorders (i.e., thyroid disease, parathyroid disease, brain tumor, uncontrolled seizure disorder, encephalitis or meningitis, etc.) that may have caused or aggravated the psychosis, and
• Use of antipsychotic medications to decrease the frequency and severity of psychotic symptoms (i.e., hallucinations of various types, delusions, thought disorganization, disorientation, agitation and hyperactivity, or profound withdrawal and/or catatonia, insomnia, etc.)

Dementia and mental retardation
Dementia is a general term for disorders that produce deterioration in memory, judgment, orientation, and ability to handle abstract data. These disorders result from degeneration in the brain itself and unlike delirium are not transient. Although there are many types of dementia, the most common forms

are Alzheimer dementia, Lewy body dementia, and vascular dementia.

Dementia is generally associated with old age (sixty years or older), but occurs in younger individuals with mental retardation or other developmental disabilities. The risk for dementia appears to be higher in individuals with mental retardation.

The association between Down syndrome (which usually causes moderate mental retardation) and Alzheimer dementia has been known since the early part of the 20th century. Not all people with Down syndrome develop Alzheimer dementia, but the risk is higher than for the general population, especially before age 50 years. The majority of people with Down syndrome do show a tendency toward deterioration in language, memory, self-care skills, and problem solving as they enter their thirties. Postmortem studies on the brains of individuals with Down syndrome over the age of 40 show a high incidence of two microscopic brain abnormalities common to Alzheimer dementia—senile plaques and neurofibrillary tangles.

Self-injurious behavior and mental retardation

Self-injurious behavior (SIB) describes a multitude of behaviors by which individuals may inflict harm on themselves. Common examples of SIB in people with retardation include head banging, slapping self, biting self, skin picking, hair pulling, placing foreign objects in any bodily orifice, gouging eyes, and ingesting harmful materials. Sometimes the behavior amounts to frank self-mutilation (i.e., the deliberate destruction of bodily tissue or parts without conscious intent to commit suicide).

When self-mutilation occurs in the general population, it is usually associated with acute psychiatric illness or with severe personality disorder. While the same can be true of self-mutilating individuals who have mental retardation, stereotypical self-mutilation can be a common feature in institutionalized people. Some authorities believe that SIB occurs predominantly in those individuals with retardation who are in residential care; other authorities counter that the pertinent issue is the severity of the mental retardation common to people who are institutionalized as compared with those who live with family or in the community. Some studies also show a greater risk for SIB in teenagers and adults as compared to young children and the elderly. Apart from two X-linked genetic disorders (Lesch-Nyhan syndrome and fragile X syndrome) that occur more commonly in males and carry a high risk for self-mutilation, SIB is approximately equally common in males and females.

In addition to the potential for long-term, permanent damage from SIB, individuals may also suffer indirectly from consequences of their behavior. Those who persist in SIB cause others around them to feel uncomfortable, helpless, frustrated, and often angry. This can result in an understandable urge by caretakers to avoid being faced with such behaviors. Neglect of self-abusive individuals can result. Studies indicate that another frequent response by caretakers may be physical abuse of the self-abuser. A third indirect result of SIB may be the exclusion of the individual from community and group activities as well as educational and occupational opportunities.

Why do individuals persist in consciously inflicting injury upon themselves? There are numerous speculations. Some authorities believe the behavior is learned and a response to the individual's internal (i.e., bodily) or external environment or both. Others suggest a neurochemical imbalance, an underlying acute or chronic condition (such as an ear infection, menstruation, or chronic constipation, especially in an individual with poor language skills who cannot relate the nature of the discomfort), chronic or unsuspected epilepsy, or a need for self-stimulation (in an individual with profound sensory deficits). Other possible causes include self-abuse as a form of communication, as a compulsion related to OCD, as a symptom of grief, or as a component of post-traumatic stress disorder.

SIBs can be resistant to treatment. Often a cause for the behavior is not apparent. When underlying conditions are discovered or suspected (e.g., ear infection, OCD, etc.), appropriate medications may diminish or even eliminate the SIB. Some SIBs with a stereotypical or compulsive quality may decrease in frequency and severity with a trial on selective serotonin reuptake inhibitors (SSRIs). Trichotillomania—the systematic plucking of individual scalp hairs causing denuded patches of scalp that may be the diameter of a quarter or even a doughnut—responds well to SSRIs. Treatment of epilepsy may eliminate some SIBs, especially when unsuspected "light" seizures cause frequent periods of irritability or confusion during which time the SIB is more likely to occur.

An important component in the management of SIBs is the behavioral response of family and other caretakers. Boredom can provoke SIB that can be suppressed by a reasonable variety of stimulation. Overstimulation can also result in SIB. In such cases, providing a quieter, more soothing environment is helpful. Sometimes self-abusive individuals (particularly those with severe to profound mental retardation) may control their own patterns of self-injury by "self-restraining." A frequently seen form of self-restraint occurs in self-abusers who sit on their hands. When they are prevented from doing so by well-meaning staff who want to help them "normalize" their behavior, self-abusers may resume their eye-gouging, skin picking, or head slapping.

Formal behavior modification programs may be devised by behavior specialists to reduce the frequency and the severity of a specific self-abusive behavior. Such programs frequently utilize rewards for appropriate behavior and loss of reward for lapse into self-abuse. Punitive measures or aversive measures should be avoided.

Occasionally, protective devices may be part of the treatment regimen, such as the use of helmets for individuals who head bang. Restrictive devices, such as hand restraints or mittens, should be used only as a last resort and only in severe situations where the potential for significant self-injury is present (i.e., when an individual persists in attempting to pluck out an eye). Seclusion is rarely safe or effective for management of self-abuse.

Psychoactive Medications

Psychoactive medications are used to minimize or eliminate disturbing symptoms of mental illness. The same medications that are effective for individuals in the general population can be effective in people with mental retardation if care is taken to minimize potential side effects such as sedation, irritability, restlessness, and dulling of thought.

Most mental retardation facilities adhere to federal and state regulations with regard to administration of psychoactive medications. The goal is to minimize the use of "chemical restraints" in favor of environmental manipulation and behavior modification.

In general, individuals with both mild mental retardation and psychiatric symptoms should receive dosages of psychoactive medications similar to those recommended for the general population. Medication should be used cautiously, however, in individuals with moderate to profound mental retardation, because they are more vulnerable to side effects of medication. In general, medications should be started at low doses and escalated slowly.

9. Research on the Future of Prevention and Treatment of Mental Retardation

The mapping of the human genome is nearing completion. Although a momentous accomplishment, this is only a first step in the dawning era of gene therapy for many of the worst human disorders, including mental retardation. Identifying single gene forms of mental retardation may pave the way to effective gene therapy for these disorders in the near future. For mental retardation syndromes resulting from complicated interactions of multiple genes, effective gene therapy must wait until the complex interplay can be unraveled. Retardation syndromes caused by environmental factors may benefit from gene therapy if damage to genes or their protein products can be minimized by replacement therapy.

Researchers anticipate that gene therapy for mental retardation may take a variety of paths resulting in improvement in diagnosis, prevention, and treatment. All will require development of new medical procedures. Evolution in philosophical, ethical, and legal concepts will also be required as researchers and clinicians raise the specter of eugenics and intensify the philosophical and legal battles concerning when human life begins.

Basic Biochemistry of the Human Genome

Deoxyribonucleic acid (DNA) is the stuff of which the human genome is built. DNA's alphabet is composed of only four characters or bases: A (adenine), C (cytosine), G (guanine), and T (thymine). In the scheme of human genetics, bases attach to one another in base pairs (bp), but adenine can combine only with thymine while guanine combines only with cytosine.

Each base in DNA is also attached to a sugar molecule and a phosphoric acid molecule to form a unit known as a nucleotide. Nucleotides are aligned by the bonds between their bp to form a double helix, a coiled structure that resembles a spiral staircase with a series of bp as the rungs. The densely-packed double helix of DNA forms a chromosome packed with genes.

Humans have roughly three billion bp that combine in series of three bp or triplets to form codons that encode for one of twenty amino acids. Combinations of bp triplets (e.g., ATTCCGGAA) produce genes that, in turn, use amino acids as building blocks to produce proteins, either structural or enzymatic, that combine to form a unique human being. When genes are altered, the proteins they encode may not function normally, thus producing genetic disorders.

Nearly all (99.9%) of humanity's genomic sequence is identical, so what produces the diversity in human traits? The difference lies in the remaining 0.1% of the human genome and appears to be due to single nucleotide polymorphisms, often called SNPs or "snips."

Found in both coding (gene) and non-coding regions of the chromosomes, SNPs are single bp variations that occur about once in every 1000 bp throughout human DNA. These minute variations can be used to track inheritance in families. In some instances, only a minimal effect is evident when a single base change occurs in a single gene. In other cases, the effect can be profound. When studied in entirety by the human genome research team, the so-named SNP map will provide the genetic interpretation of unique differences, the genetic predisposition for certain diseases, and the genetic basis for individualized responses to specific treatment modalities.

The SNP Consortium (TSC) is a public-private partnership of academic institutions, pharmaceutical companies, and charitable organizations that guides the cataloging of SNPs. TSC works collaboratively with the Human Genome Project (HGP). By the fall of 2002, TSC had published more than 1.2 million SNPs and categorized an estimated 1.8 million.

What Is Gene Therapy?

Gene therapy is a technique for correcting defective genes. As abnormal gene patterns producing specific mental retardation syndromes are identified, the possibility of correcting genetic defects and eliminating the pathology becomes more promising.

Four approaches to gene therapy are currently being studied. The most common approach is the insertion of a normal gene into a nonspecific location within the genome. The normal gene theoretically becomes active and replaces the nonfunctional gene. A second method involves removal of an abnormal gene, replacing it with a normal gene through a process known as homologous recombination (e.g., the exchange of pieces of DNA between pairs of similar chromosomes). A third method is the repair of an abnormal gene through selective reverse mutation, thus returning the gene to normal function. Yet another approach involves the regulation of a specific gene so that its level of activity can be enhanced or diminished.

Most gene therapy research presently focuses on replacement of an defective gene with a normal one. To do this, a normal gene must be ferried into human target cells. Currently, the most common method of transport involves using a virus that has itself been genetically altered to carry normal human DNA into the genes of human cells. The normal gene then becomes incorporated into the chromosomes of target cells and begins producing the required normal protein.

Non-viral methods of introducing therapeutic DNA into target cells are also being studied. The simplest is the direct introduction of DNA into the nucleus of target cells, but this approach is limited because it can be used only with certain tissues and requires large amounts of DNA.

A second non-viral method involves the creation of a liposome, a minute sphere formed of phospholipid (fatty acid with attached phosphate) with a fluid core. The liposome is capable of passing through the protective cell wall, carrying within it the therapeutic DNA.

Another non-viral approach involves chemically linking therapeutic DNA to a molecule that will bind to cell wall receptors and be engulfed into the target cells.

A fourth approach is the introduction a 47th artificial chromosome carrying the needed gene into the target cell. The artificial chromosome coexists with the standard 46 chromosomes and ideally does not affect their function except for correcting the gene abnormality. The problem with this method is that it requires a large molecule of DNA that is difficult to deliver to the nucleus of target cells.

Current Status of Gene Therapy Research

Gene therapy remains experimental at this point. Experimental trials, first begun in 1990, have not yet proven very successful. Some have had lethal results. In 1999, Jesse

Gelsinger, an 18-year old who was participating in a gene therapy trial, died from multiple organ failure within four days of beginning gene treatments. His death was apparently the result of a severe immune response to the transport virus used to ferry DNA into his cells.

In January 2003, the U.S. Food and Drug Administration (FDA) placed a temporary halt on all gene therapy trials using retroviruses as the DNA carrier into blood stem cells after two young children developed a leukemia-like condition following gene therapy for an X-linked severe immune deficiency known as "bubble baby syndrome." Gene therapy research using retroviruses in the U.S. is currently on hold awaiting FDA approval, but resumption with safeguards in place is anticipated.

Complicating gene therapy research is the difficulty in ensuring that therapeutic DNA inserted into target cells will be long-lived, stable, functional, and able to integrate into the human genome without causing serious side effects. Anytime foreign material is introduced into human tissues, there is a risk of activating the immune system. The immune response may limit the effectiveness of gene therapy, especially if the treatment requires repeated insertions of therapeutic DNA. There is also an obvious risk that the viruses used in most gene therapy studies may prove toxic, cause severe immune responses, or even recover their ability to cause disease in the patient.

The Future of Gene Therapy and Mental Retardation

As human genome research identifies specific genes or combinations of genes that cause mental retardation syndromes, the diagnosis of affected individuals will become more precise and, in turn, allow more accurate genetic counseling for couples planning pregnancies, especially those couples who have family members with mental retardation.

Genetic counseling is a process that provides patients and families with information about genetic disorders that may "run in the family." The information includes the risk for individuals developing the disorder as well as the risk for passing the disorder on to subsequent generations. The information allows people to make informed decisions regarding the welfare of themselves and their family, especially with regard to decisions about pregnancy. This benefit triggers legal and ethical concerns if a couple chooses to take a chance on pregnancy despite the risk of passing on abnormal genetic material. Lab tests can already identify some hereditary disorders in unborn children, but in the near future intrauterine tests will be more accurate, screen for many additional disorders, and be effective earlier in the mother's pregnancy. Diagnostic advances have already outpaced advances in treatment, thus intensifying ethical, legal, and philosophical arguments related to abortion.

Researchers anticipate that understanding the human genome will provide the means for preventing some forms of mental retardation other than through abortion of abnormal fetuses. Research is already under way into methods of replacing or masking abnormal genes in utero so that normal development of the nervous system can occur. The end result of preventive measures will be to correct abnormalities before damage is done to the nervous system of the fetus.

The goal of treatment in individuals diagnosed after birth will be either to minimize the severity of mental retardation syndromes or to cure them (i.e., eliminate all symptoms of retardation in individuals and their offspring). Gene therapy holds promise in both areas. Introduction of corrective genetic material into the genome of an individual with mental retardation (the earlier, the better) should alleviate or totally correct some of the pathology associated with mental retardation syndromes.

The same result may be accomplished by administering specific enzymes that are missing or inactive due to abnormal genes rather than by introducing the genes themselves. How are these therapeutic enzymes to be identified and created? After the individual genes of the human genome are identified, further research will be needed to identify the structural proteins or the enzymes the genes produce and the series of steps that follow to produce a normal human being.

The success of gene therapy in eliminating mental retardation will be limited by the multiple causes of such syndromes. As noted above, retardation disorders caused by single gene abnormalities are the best candidates for gene therapy. Unfortunately, the majority of mental retardation syndromes are caused by variations of multiple genes and/or environmental factors. Gene therapy for these disorders will be difficult to achieve and, at best, will probably serve to minimize symptoms, not to cure the disorder.

Two retardation syndromes closely studied for gene therapy include Lesch-Nyhan syndrome and phenylketonuria (see chapter 1). Animal models of these disorders allow current gene therapy research to progress before contemplating human trials.

Down syndrome, the most common chromosomal abnormality causing mental retardation, presents a problem for current methods of gene therapy research. An extra chromosome 21 is known to be present in the disorder, but an analysis of the specific number and locations of genes involved is not yet complete.

An Example: Fragile X Syndrome

Fragile X syndrome provides a window into ongoing research related to the origins of specific mental retardation syndromes. As described in chapter 1, fragile X syndrome is the second most common cause of inherited mental retardation after Down syndrome. The disorder is inherited in an X-linked recessive pattern so that the condition is twice as common in males as in females. Recent research has identified the defective gene (FMR1) on the long arm of the X chromosome.

Misdiagnosis of fragile X syndrome is common. As a result of human genome research, diagnosis of this single gene disorder may soon be more precise. Recent studies indicate that the defective FMR1 gene contains excessive numbers of CGG triplet repeats, typically more than two hundred. The defective gene codes for the mRNA (messenger ribonucleic acid) binding protein.

The DNA in FMR1 varies in length among individuals depending on the numbers of CGG repeats. Among some men and women, the varying length constitutes a "premutation" that does not cause symptoms of fragile X syndrome. These individuals have relatively fewer triplet repeats and thus a shorter length of DNA.

Over successive generations, the premutation is passed to children with the possibility of adding more CGG repeats so that the likelihood of a full mutation becomes greater with each generation. When the DNA is lengthened beyond a certain point, its protein-producing capability is lost. This full gene mutation presents as an individual with fragile X syndrome. To some degree, the severity of the syndrome may be related to the number of nucleotide repeats in FMR1: The greater the number of triplet repeats, the more severe the pathology.

Diagnosis of fragile X syndrome can now be confirmed through detection of the full mutation of the FMR1 gene. All women of child-bearing age who have a child diagnosed with the syndrome are carriers for FMR1 gene expansion and are at increased risk of successive reproductive impairments. Genetic testing can confirm the diagnosis. Genetic counseling is advised.

Likewise, genetic testing may be considered for people of either gender who have mental retardation, developmental delays or autism, relatives with undiagnosed mental retardation, and carriers of fragile X syndrome.

The National Institute of Child Health and Human Development reports that molecular genetic screening and subsequent implantation of syndrome-free, in vitro-fertilized embryos may be a reality in the near future. Animal models are presently being studied.

Researchers at Columbia University recently created transgenic mouse lines that harbor some genetic defects similar to those causing genetic disorders in humans, including fragile X syndrome. These will provide animal models for both short term treatment methodologies and long term genetic therapies for fragile X syndrome. Thus far, researchers working with a transgenic mouse line have isolated a chemical known as MPEP that blocks a receptor designated in the synthesis of a specific protein. Some correlation may exist between blocked receptor action and behavioral improvement in the transgenic mouse lines. Treatment advances along this line will be limited until more is learned about the biological basis of fragile X syndrome and how DNA nucleotide expansions occur on the long arm of the X chromosome.

Ethical Questions and Gene Therapy

The science of genetics has progressed rapidly since the 1800s when the Austrian monk Mendel recorded his observations on cross-pollinating peas. As biological knowledge mushrooms, will ethical considerations keep pace? Our ability to balance thirst for knowledge with ethical considerations will be of primary importance in the coming decades.

As genetic research continues its rapid advance, society must define normality and disability while being cautious about who makes the determination. We must decide whether normality for all is a desired outcome or if genetic diversity is more desirable. We must determine whether it is ethical to alter individual germlines (i.e., to prevent a trait from being passed on to future generations) or turn instead to somatic gene therapy in which the procedure will have to be repeated in future generations.

Society already has access to in utero screening for some genetic disorders and thus is faced with ethical considerations related to termination of pregnancy. As human genome research allows us to read the blueprint for each individual, there will be a temptation to pre-select "desirable" traits in the formation of human embryos and to "deselect" undesirable embryos. Many people argue that this will bring an end to tragic hereditary disabilities. It also may reintroduce the specter of eugenics.

Eugenics, in its more benign interpretation, is a science that investigates methods of improving the genetic composition of the human race. In its more virulent forms, eugenics has become the pseudo-science justifying bigotry and racism in Europe, Great Britain, the United States, Scandinavia, and Asia. In its perverted form, eugenics haunted disadvantaged groups (e.g., European Jews as well as individuals with mental illness and those with mental retardation) during the first half of the 20th century, when Hitler sought to "cleanse" Europe. During the same period, mental institutions in Europe and the United States sterilized patients with mental disorders.

Human genome research and ethics must deal directly with the advisability of building human beings to specifications. Society may wish to eliminate genetic disabilities, but does it want to develop "cookie cutter" people with similar skills, mental abilities, and physical appearance? What genius may be lost if we "correct" all future humans toward the "high norm," thus eliminating diversity and unique promise? Under such a system, it is doubtful that Albert Einstein would have made his appearance, as his genius appears to have been related to his abnormal brain structure.

Society will also need to deal with the expense of gene therapy. The research and the procedures themselves will be costly. Ethical considerations must be included in decisions about who will receive the benefit of gene therapy and who will bear the cost-and who will make these determinations.

Appendix A

Who May Benefit from Genetic Counseling? (Center for Medical Genetics)

- Parents of a child born with a genetic disorder, birth defect, or chromosome abnormality
- Couples who have experienced repeated pregnancy losses or difficulty becoming pregnant
- Children with developmental delay and unusual features
- Individuals who fail to develop secondary sexual characteristics
- Children with short stature that is unusual for the family
- Women or their infants who have been exposed to a medication, drug, radiation, or other environmental agent
- People with a family history of a birth defect or genetic disease
- Couples with older maternal or paternal age
- Individuals of certain ethnic groups at increased risk for genetic disorders (African Americans, Ashkenazic Jews, Mediterraneans)
- Individuals interested in prenatal diagnosis
- Individuals with a family history of cancer

Appendix B

Milestones of Human Development

Birth
- Aware of light and dark (closes eyelids in bright light)
- Can turn head from side to side when prone on a surface

4 weeks
- Eyes follow large, conspicuously moving objects
- Makes throaty sounds
- Able to lift head above surface

2 months
- Smiles when social contact is made
- Produces sounds with evident pleasure on social contact

3 months
- Eyes and head follow moving object
- Enjoys light objects and bright colors
- Smiles spontaneously
- Head turns toward sound
- Head does not lag when infant is pulled to an upright position
- Able to maintain control of head when upright without head bobbing
- Able to raise head and chest from surface when prone
- Reaches for objects
- Holds rattle placed in hand
- Begins to hold head erect
- Squeals and babbles (initial sounds are vowels)

4 months
- Inspects own hands
- Makes guttural sounds
- Able to laugh aloud at pleasurable social contact

• May show displeasure by change of expression (fussing or crying) when pleasurable contact is withdrawn
• Grasps objects and brings them to midline (often to mouth to explore)

5 months
• Shows interest in objects more than three feet away
• Enjoys being supported in an upright posture
• Attracted to objects presented on a plane surface

6 months
• Begins babbling with active vocalization
• Can maintain voluntary visual fixation on a stationary object even in the presence of competing moving stimuli
• Reaches with one hand to grasp object
• Begins to differentiate between familiar persons and strangers
• Shows a preference for the person giving most of the care
• Transfers toy from hand to hand
• Can pick up small object
• Reaches out with arms to be picked up
• Able to roll over
• Able to change the orientation of the entire body in order to extend a hand toward a desired large object (such as a rattle)
• Able to sit alone
• Becomes increasingly interested in own legs
• Able to support weight upon extended legs when pulled upright

7 months
• Imitates speech sounds
• Shows response to the emotional tone of social contacts, including response to changes in

the facial expressions of those in the familiar environment
- Able to pivot in the prone position in order to pursue an object within reach

8 months
- Complains when mother leaves room
- Becomes attentive at the sound of own name

9 months
- Says "dada" or "mama" but without meaning
- Can pull self erect (holding on)
- Can sit on floor with back straight and without rolling over
- Imitates sounds
- Feeds self cracker or cookie with ease
- Depth perception begins to develop
- Picks up small object with thumb and one finger
- Begins to creep or crawl (some normal babies never crawl and go directly from creeping to walking)
- Begins to stand steady for a short time so long as both hands are held
- Begins to take tentative first steps when both hands are held
- Becomes less dependent upon the physical presence of the mother, because is increasingly able to follow her around
- Learns that being out of sight does not mean that object is not available (begins to enjoy peek-a-boo games)
- Likes to play pat-a-cake
- Waves goodbye

12 months
- Walks, with one hand held
- Cruises, if holding onto furniture
- May take one or two independent steps

- Says one or two words (besides "mama" and "dada")
- Repeats a few single words
- Gives toy on request

15 months
- Walks independently with feet wide apart
- Has four- to six-word vocabulary
- Creeps upstairs
- Climbs stairs one step at a time with one hand held
- Builds tower of two cubes
- Pats pictures in book
- Casts objects in play
- Explores environment

18 months
- Walks alone although balance is unsteady
- Runs stiffly
- Turns pages of book, two or three at a time
- Has vocabulary of 8 to 10 words, including names (may not be complete or pronounced properly but are clearly meaningful)

24 months
- Runs well, no falling
- Turns pages of book singly
- Uses three-word sentences (not usually complete or grammatically correct)
- Vowels uttered correctly
- Begins use of pronouns
- Has approximately 270-word vocabulary
- Refers to self by name
- Can follow a few simple directions
- Says variety of everyday words heard in home and neighborhood
- Can identify several parts of body
- Able to verbalize toilet needs

30 months
- Knows full name
- Can say or sing short rhymes or songs
- Can identify some simple objects by use (cup, shoe, car)
- Begins to use personal pronoun "I"
- Unbuttons front buttons

36 months
- Can copy a circle
- Can copy a straight line
- Alternates feet going upstairs
- Rides tricycle using pedals
- Feeds self at mealtime, spills little
- Uses plurals
- Knows own gender
- Repeats six to seven syllables
- Speaks in complete sentences some of the time, usually up to four-word phrases
- Has approximately 900-word vocabulary

42 months
- Understands a few prepositions ("put ball on chair")
- Washes and dries face and hands
- Takes off shoes and jacket
- Copies drawing of a cross
- Can carry out a simple request

48 months
- Names one or two colors
- Can carry out a sequence of two simple directions
- Answers correctly "what do we have houses for?"
- Answers correctly "what do we have books for?"
- Answers correctly "what do we do when we are thirsty?"
- Uses five-word phrases or sentences

- Has approximately 1540-word vocabulary
- Alternates feet going downstairs

5 years
- Knows four or five colors
- Copies a triangle
- Prints a few letters
- Uses pronouns correctly
- Copies a square
- Can count four objects
- Names penny, nickel, quarter
- Runs and turns without losing balance
- May stand on one leg for at least ten seconds
- Can hop on one foot
- Can toilet alone (occasionally needs assistance with wiping)
- Dresses self except for tying

6 years
- Has concepts of simple numbers
- Draws a person with neck, hands, and clothes
- Can count to 30
- Speaks in six- to seven-word phrases
- Has approximately 2560-word vocabulary
- Can catch ball
- Skips smoothly
- Knows right hand from left
- Draws recognizable man with at least eight details
- Can describe favorite television show in some detail
- Does simple chores at home (such as taking out garbage or drying silverware)
- Good motor ability but little awareness of dangers

7 years
- Answers correctly "what makes a sail boat move?"

- Can copy a diamond
- Can count five digits
- Ties shoestrings
- Repeats five numbers in succession
- Can count by 5's
- Draws a man with twelve details
- Reads several one-syllable words (My, dog, cat, see, boy, girl)
- Uses pencil for printing name
- Knows what day of the week it is
- Has learned to group objects together in classes

8 years
- Knows the days of the week
- Counts backward from 20 to 1
- Does simple subtraction
- Has learned that objects can be reversed (i.e., 2 + 2 = 4 but also 4 − 2 = 2)
- Has adult proficiency in language
- Can read simple paragraphs

9 years
- Makes change with coins
- Knows the months in correct order
- Repeats four numbers backward
- Can do simple multiplication and division

12 years
- Has learned about constancy in amounts despite inconstancy of shape (same amount of water will appear at different levels in a tall, thin glass and a short, fat glass)
- Able to do advanced multiplication and division

Adolescence
- Learns to handle abstract thoughts
- Learns to reason
- Learns to formulate hypotheses and to test them in reality and thought

Appendix C

Selected Federal Legislation and Regulations Pertinent to Mental Retardation

1963 Public Law 88-164, The Mental Retardation Research Facilities and Community Mental Health Centers Construction Act

Authorizes grants for the construction of 14 centers for research on mental retardation and related aspects of human development.

Mental Retardation Research Centers (MRRCs) provide greater visibility for research in mental retardation within the larger research community. They successfully attract basic and clinical research scientists to address the multifaceted programs in mental retardation and developmental disabilities. Core grants both facilitate program coordination and support central research facilities. Funds for specific research projects that use these core facilities come from independent sources including the National Institute of Child Health and Human Development (NICHD), other NIH institutes, other federal agencies, state governments, and private foundations.

1968, Public Law 90-284, Fair Housing Act, Title VIII of the Civil Rights Act, as amended

Prohibits discrimination in the sale, rental, and financing of housing and in other housing-related transactions based on race, color, national origin, religion, sex, familial status. This prohibition includes children under the age of 18 living with parents or legal custodians, pregnant women, and people securing custody of children under the age of 18 and people with disabilities.

Under the Fair Housing Act, it is unlawful to discriminate in any aspect of selling, renting, or denying housing because of an individual's disability. Owners are further required to make reasonable exceptions in their housing policies so as to afford equal housing opportunities to those with disabilities.

Complaints about housing issues may be filed with United States Housing and Urban Development at the website, www.hud.gov

1968, Public Law 90-480, Architectural Barriers Act (ABA)

An increasing awareness of problems faced by many Americans encountering accessibility barriers caused Congress to evaluate issues in 1965. In September of that year, Congress created the National Commission on Architectural Barriers to Rehabilitation of the Handicapped. The Commission's charge was to determine to the extent to which architectural barriers prevented access to public facilities, report on what was being done to eliminate barriers, and propose measures to eliminate and prevent barriers.

The Commission's report, issued in June 1968, laid the groundwork for the Architectural Barriers Act of 1968 (ABA). This law requires accessibility in buildings and facilities designed, built, or modified with federal monies or leased by federal agencies. Accessibility standards are applied to all building structures, paths of travel, parking space allocation, ramps, counter heights, restroom facilities and related public spaces.

Several years after the ABA became law, Congress observed that compliance had been uneven and that no initiatives to create federal design standards for accessibility were under way. The concept of such an agency began to take shape as Congress considered the Rehabilitation Act of 1973. Section 502 of this law created the Access Board, originally named the Architectural and Transportation Barriers Compliance Board. The Board was charged with ensuring federal agency compliance with the ABA and proposing solutions to the environmental barriers problems addressed in the ABA.

The Access Board is an independent federal agency devoted to accessibility for people with disabilities. It operates with about 30 staff and a governing board of representatives from federal departments and public members appointed by the President. The Access Board publishes Access Currents, a bi-monthly newsletter available in electronic format. The newsletter provides an ongoing update of activities for which the Board is responsible, such as the changes to ADA and ABA accessibility guidelines. The newsletter can be found at the Board's website, under "About the Board: Services." See www.access-board.gov/

1973, Public Law 93-112, The Rehabilitation Act, as amended, Section 501, 29 U.S.C. § 791, Section 503, 29 U.S.C. § 793, Section 504, 29 U.S.C. § 794 and Section 508, 29 U.S.C. § 794d

The Rehabilitation Act prohibits discrimination on the basis of disability in programs conducted by federal agencies, in programs receiving federal financial assistance, in federal employment, and in the employment practices of federal contractors. Its standards mirror those of the ADA. Passage of The Rehabilitation Act of 1973, as amended, and its subsequent sections are cited as the greatest achievement of the disability rights movement and a precursor to the Americans with Disabilities Act of 1990 (ADA). This legislation also established the Architectural and Transportation Barriers Compliance Board, now the Access Board, to enforce the Architectural Barriers Act of 1968.

This rehabilitative statute, particularly Title V and Section 504, prohibited discrimination by programs receiving federal funds against "otherwise qualified handicapped" individuals. In so doing, disability rights advocates and advocacy organizations found a weapon with which they would combat anti-disability activities. Litigation that followed its passage conceptualized now-familiar issues such as "reasonable modification," "reasonable accommodation," and "undue burden." Such concepts formed the framework of the ADA. Section 501 directed federal agencies to develop affirmative action programs for hiring, placement and advancement of people with disabilities. Section 502 established the Architectural and Transportation Barriers Compliance Board (ATBCB) to ensure compliance with the Architectural Barriers Act of 1968, pursue methods to eliminate transportation barriers, and research methods for accessible housing. Section 503 required that contractors with the United States develop and use affirmative action to employ qualified people with disabilities. Section 504 stated: "No otherwise qualified handicapped individual in the United States shall, solely by reason of his handicap, be excluded from the participation in, be denied the benefits of, or be subjected to discrimination under any program or activity receiving federal financial assistance."

According to the National Council on Disability, the Rehabilitation Act joins with the Civil Rights Act of 1964 as "twin philosophical pillars" for subsequent legislative gains. Section 504, particularly, moved disability policy from a welfare mentality to a right-to-access concept. First, Section 504 couched discriminatory practices in terms of illegal actions. Secondly, the growing disability rights community used this section as a battering ram when seeking regulatory requirements after passage. Finally, legal standards established by this section became foundational to the ADA.

Section 508 establishes requirements for electronic and information technology developed, maintained, procured or used by the federal government. Section 508 requires federal electronic and information technology to be accessible to people with disabilities, including employees and members of the public. An accessible information technology system is one that can be operated in a variety of ways and does not rely on a single sense or ability of the user. For example, a system that provides output only in visual format may not be accessible to people with visual impairments and a system that provides output only in audio format may not be accessible to people who are deaf or hard of hearing. Some individuals with disabilities may need accessibility-related software or peripheral devices in order to use systems that comply with Section 508. For additional references to the Rehabilitation Act, see its Section 501, 29 U.S.C. § 791, Section 503, 29 U.S.C. § 793, Section 504, 29 U.S.C. § 794 and Section 508, 29 U.S.C. § 794d.

1975, Public Law 94-142, the *Education for All Handicapped Children Act (EHA)*

Regarded by many authorities as setting the foundation for today's disability rights principles. P.L. 94-142 asserted full, free, and appropriate rights for all children with disabilities. Subsequent reauthorizations mandated educational services for children from birth through 21 years of age. The EAHCA has been reauthorized several times, with a variety of amendments governing issues such as early intervention services for infants and toddlers, attorney's fees for families who successfully challenge their children's special education programs, the addition of certain services (such as transition plans for older students and assistive technology), the addition of certain disabilities that could qualify children for special education (such as traumatic brain injury and autism), and changes in nomenclature to recognize society's newfound use of the word "disability" in place of "handicap." In the 1990 reauthorization, the name of the statute was changed from EAHCA to IDEA.

1975, Public Law 100-146, The Protection and Advocacy for Persons with Developmental Disabilities (PADD) Program, The Developmental Disabilities Assistance and Bill of Rights (DD) Act, Part C. [1994 amendments to the DD Act expanded the system to include a Native American P&A program.]

Protection and advocacy systems are required by the Act to pursue legal, administrative and other appropriate remedies to protect and advocates for the rights of individuals with developmental disabilities under all applicable federal and state laws. The Administration for Children Youth and Families, Administration on Developmental Disabilities (ADD) administers the PADD program. The governor in each state designates an agency to be the P&A system and provides assurance that the system is and will remain independent of any service provider. Information about states' Protection and Advocacy Systems may be located through directory assistance or on the national website, www.protectionandadvocacy.org. Website addresses and other contact information may be referenced in the Resources section of this book.

The Client Assistance Program (CAP) was established as a mandatory program by the 1984 Amendments to the Rehabilitation Act. Each state's system pursues legal, administrative and other appropriate remedies to protect and promote rights of individuals under all applicable federal and state laws.

The Protection and Advocacy for Individuals with Mental Illness (PAIMI) Program was established in 1986. Each state has a PAIMI program which receives funding from the national Center for Mental Health Services. Agencies are mandated to (1) protect and advocate for the rights of people with mental illness and (2) investigate reports of abuse and neglect in facilities that care for or treat individuals with mental illness.

Agencies provide advocacy services or conduct investigations to address issues which arise during transportation or admission to the time of residency in, or within 90 days after discharge from, such facilities. The system designated to serve as the PADD program in each state and territory is also responsible for operating the PAIMI program. Substance Abuse and Mental Health Services Administration, Center for Mental Health Services (CMHS) administers the PAIMI program.

The Protection and Advocacy for Individual Rights (PAIR) Program was established by Congress as a national program under the Rehabilitation Act in 1993. PAIR programs were established to protect and advocate for the legal and human rights of persons with disabilities. Although PAIR is funded at a lower level than PADD and PAIMI, it represents an important component of a comprehensive system to advocate for the rights of all persons with disabilities. The system designated to serve as the PADD program in each state and territory is also responsible for operating the PAIR program. Office of Special Education and Rehabilitative Services, Rehabilitation Services Administration (RSA) administers PAIR.

1980, Public Law 96-247, Civil Rights for Institutionalized Persons Act (CRIPA)

The Civil Rights of Institutionalized Persons Act (CRIPA) authorizes the U.S. Attorney General to investigate conditions of confinement at State and local government institutions such as prisons, jails, pretrial detention centers, juvenile correctional facilities, publicly operated nursing homes and institutions for people with psychiatric or developmental disabilities. CRIPA does not cover individuals confined to private entities. The Act's purpose is to allow the Attorney General to uncover and correct widespread deficiencies that seriously jeopardize the health and safety of residents of institutions. The Attorney

General does not have authority under CRIPA to investigate isolated incidents or to represent individual institutionalized persons.

The Attorney General may initiate civil lawsuits where there is reasonable cause to believe that conditions are "egregious or flagrant," that they are subjecting residents to "grievous harm," and that they are part of a "pattern or practice" of resistance to residents' full enjoyment of constitutional or federal rights, including title II of the ADA and section 504 of the Rehabilitation Act. For more information, contact Special Litigation Section, Civil Rights Division, U.S. Department of Justice. www.doj.ocr.gov

1984, Public Law 98-435. Voting Accessibility for the Elderly and Handicapped Act

The Voting Accessibility for the Elderly and Handicapped Act of 1984 generally requires polling places across the United States to be physically accessible to people with disabilities for federal elections. Where no accessible location is available to serve as a polling place, a political subdivision must provide an alternate means of casting a ballot on the day of the election. This law also requires states to make available registration and voting aids for disabled and elderly voters, including information by telecommunications devices for the deaf (TDDs) which are also known as teletypewriters (TTYs). For more information, contact Voting Section, Civil Rights Division, U.S. Department of Justice. See www.usdoj.gov/crt/voting

1986, Public Law 99-147, Amended the Education for All Handicapped Children Act (EHA), as amended, Part H

Established the Handicapped Infants and Toddlers Program. Under these amendments, states were required to develop and implement a statewide interagency system of interventions for children with disabilities, children at risk for disabilities and their families. Congressional amendments during the 1990s further modified the original law. Under 1997 IDEA modifications, Part H became Part C.

1986, Public Law 99-435, Air Carrier Access Act

Under the Air Carrier Access Act, air carriers are prohibited from discrimination in air transportation against qualified individuals with physical and/or mental impairments by domestic and foreign air carriers. It applies only to air carriers that provide regularly scheduled services for hire to the public. Requirements address a wide range of issues including boarding assistance and certain accessibility features in newly built aircraft and new or altered airport facilities. People may enforce rights under the Air Carrier Access Act by filing a complaint with the U.S. Department of Transportation, or by bringing a lawsuit in federal court. For more information or to file a complaint, contact the Aviation Consumer Protection Division, U.S. Department of Transportation. See www.dot.gov/

1990, Public Law 104-327, American with Disabilities Act (ADA)

The ADA prohibits discrimination on the basis of disability in employment, State and local government, public accommodations, commercial facilities, transportation, and telecommunications. It also applies to the United States Congress.

To be protected by the ADA, one must have a disability or have a relationship or association with an individual with a disability. An individual with a disability is defined by the ADA as a person who has a physical or mental impairment that substantially limits one or more major life activities, a person who has a history or record of such an impairment, or a person who is perceived by others as having such an impairment. The ADA does not identify by name all impairments that are covered by this law.

The U.S. Department of Justice provides free ADA materials. Printed materials may be ordered by calling the ADA Information Line (1-800-514-0301 (Voice) or 1-800-514-0383 (TDD). Publications are available in standard print as well as large print, audiotape, Braille, and computer disk for people with disabilities. Automated service is available 24 hours a day for recorded information and to order publications. To order a publication by fax, call the *ADA Information Line* and follow the directions for placing a fax order. When prompted to enter the document number, enter the specific number from the following publication list.

1996, Public Law 104-104, Telecommunications Act

The Telecommunications Act, a major revision of the Communications Act of 1937, requires manufacturers of telecommunications equipment and providers of telecommunications services to ensure that such equipment and services are accessible to and usable by people with disabilities, if readily achievable. The amendments include a broad range of products and services: telephones, cell phones, pagers, call-waiting and operator services that were inaccessible to many users with disabilities.

2000, Public Law 106-402, Developmental Disabilities Assistance and Bill of Rights Act of 2000

Disability law is largely regulated by the Americans with Disabilities Act (ADA) of 1990. This Act prohibits discrimination against individuals with disabilities in employment, housing, education, and access to public services. The ADA defines a disability as any of the following: 1. "a physical or mental impairment that substantially limits one or more of the major life activities of the individual," 2. "a record of such impairment," or 3. "being regarded as having such an impairment."

While alcoholism is included as a disability, other socially undesirable behavior is excluded from the Act. For example, sexual behavior disorders like pedophilia, transvestism, compulsive gambling, and pyromania are all excluded. The ADA, however, does not list all impairments covered. The ADA further requires that reasonable accommodation be made so as to provide individuals with disabilities equal opportunities.

Agencies and departments charged with enforcement of the ADA include the Equal Employment Opportunity Commission (EEOC) and the Department of Justice. States may pass disability statutes so long as they are consistent with the ADA.

Appendix D

Selected Governmental and Organizational Resources

Governmental Resources

Americans with Disabilities Act Home Page
www.ada.gov

Clearinghouse on Disability Information
U.S. Department of Education
330 C Street, S.W.
Room 3132, Switzer Building
Washington, D.C. 20202-2524
Phone: 202-205-8241
TDD: 202-205-4208

National Human Genome Research Institute
www.genome.gov/Education
The National Human Genome Research Institute
(NHGRI), formerly the National Center for Human Genome
Research (NCHGR), was established in 1989 to carry out the
role of the National Institutes of Health (NIH) in the International Human Genome Project (HGP). The HGP was
developed in collaboration with the United States Department
of Energy (DOE). In 1990, HGP began its work to map the
human genome. In 1997 the United States Department of
Health and Human Services (DHHS) renamed NCHGR the
National Human Genome Research Institute (NHGRI).

National Institute of Health, National Library of Medicine
www.nlm.nih.gov/medlineplus/birthdefects

MEDLINE Plus, a web-based health information resource of the National Library of Medicine, contains topics by broad groups, drug information, dictionaries, medical encyclopedias, articles, links to other organizations, and interactive health tutorials. Disability-specific information relative to birth defects is located at this site. Materials are available in Spanish.

United States Department of Health and Human Services, Administration for Children and Families, Administration on Developmental Disabilities
www.acf.dhhs.gov

The Administration on Developmental Disabilities (ADD) oversees national developmental disabilities programs that are carried out primarily at the state level. A fourth program addresses issues that are of concern to citizens across the nation. The ADD funds:

- University Centers of Excellence (UCEs)
- State Council on Developmental Disabilities (SCDD)
- Protection & Advocacy, Inc. (PAI)
- Projects of National Significance (PNS)

Protection and Advocacy for Persons with Developmental Disabilities (PADD) Program
www.protectionandadvocacy.org

State Children's Health Insurance Program Consumer Information
www.dhhs.gov/children
insurekidsnow.gov

The Centers for Disease Control and Prevention (CDC), National Center for Birth Defects and Developmental Disabilities

www.cdc.gov/ncbddd/dd

The Centers for Disease Control and Prevention (CDC) is recognized as the lead federal agency for protecting the health and safety of people—at home and abroad—providing credible information to enhance health decisions, and promoting health through strong partnerships. CDC serves as the national focus for developing and applying disease prevention and control, environmental health, and health promotion and education activities designed to improve the health of the people of the United States. CDC, located in Atlanta, Georgia, is an agency of the United States Department of Health and Human Services.

The National Center on Birth Defects and Developmental Disabilities (NCBDDD) at the Centers for Disease Control and Prevention (CDC) seeks to promote optimal fetal, infant, and child development; prevent birth defects and childhood developmental disabilities; and enhance the quality of life and prevent secondary conditions among children, adolescents, and adults who are living with a disability.

United States Department of Education, National Institute on Disability and Rehabilitation Research

ABLEDATA

www.abledata.com

A program sponsored by the National Institute on Disability and Rehabilitation Research. Web-based information on assistive technology resources.

Families and Advocates Partnership for Education (FAPE)

www.fape.org

The Families and Advocates Partnership for Education (FAPE) project is a strong partnership that aims to improve the educational outcomes for children with disabilities. It links families, advocates, and self-advocates to communicate the new focus of the Individuals with Disabilities Education Act (IDEA). The project represents the needs of 6 million children with disabilities. FAPE is one of four projects funded by the U.S. Department of Education to reach parents, administrators, service providers, and policymakers nationwide with information about implementing IDEA '97. The FAPE website contains updates on the 1999 reauthorization of IDEA and user manuals for parents and professionals.

United States Department of Energy, Human Genome Project
www.ornl.gov/TechResources/Human_Genome
This website is the Human Genome Project Information page. The site contains education, program goals and timelines, research, ethical, legal and social issues. Links to the Human Genome Project provide additional references.

United States Department of Justice
Guide to Disability Rights Information
www.usdoj.gov/crt/ada/cguide

Organizational Resources

Auburn University, School of Education, Administration
www.auburn.edu/administration/aaeeo/majorlaws/
constitution
Website on major constitutional laws and disability rights.

Autism Society of America
www.autism-society.org
7910 Woodmont Ave., Ste. 300
Bethesda, MD 20814-3067

Phone: 301-657-0881
Toll-free: 800-3AUTISM (328-8476)
Fax: 301-657-0869
Email: info@autism-society.org
Founded in 1965, the Autism Society of America (ASA) provides information and education and support for persons with autism. Services provided: information dissemination, referral service. Disability(s) served: physical, speech.

Awesome Library—Mental Retardation
www.awesomelibrary.org
See Library—Special Education—Mental Retardation

Breast Health Access for Women with Disabilities
www.bhawd.org
Parent organization is based in California. Their new publication, *Table Manners and Beyond*, is targeted to OB-GYN physicians. Information is helpful to women with mental retardation, their physicians or caregivers. Website has links to Women with Disabilities, providing other organizations with additional information.

Closing the Gap
www.closingthegap.com/index
Website that focuses on educational needs, including computer technology in special education and rehabilitation. Maintains a newsletter and links to other disability-related organizations and resources.

Disability Resources
www.disabilityresources.org/index
A nonprofit organization, Disability Resources contains publications, information on free or inexpensive publications

and materials and disability-specific topics. Includes annotated hyperlinked bibliographies on topics such as sexuality and mental retardation.

Down Syndrome Health Issues
www.ds-health.com
Website authored by pediatrician who is a parent of a son with Down syndrome. Essays of general interest. Includes archives from November 1997.

Education News
www.educationnews.org/mental_retardation.htm
Website of education news with special link emphasis on mental retardation. Site includes linkages to other organizations, publications and articles of interest to parents or professional educators.

Epilepsy Foundation of America
www.efa.org
4351 Garden City Drive
Landover, MD 20785
Phone: 301-459-3700
Toll Free: 800-332-1000

ERIC Clearinghouse Resources
www.ericec.org
The ERIC Clearinghouse on Disabilities and Gifted Education (ERIC EC)
The Council for Exceptional Children
1110 N. Glebe Rd.
Arlington, VA 22201-5704
Toll-free: 800-328-0272
E-mail: ericec@cec.sped.org

Family Voices
www.familyvoices.org
Family Voices National Office
3411 Candelaria NE, Suite M
Albuquerque, NM 87107
Phone: 505-872-4774
Fax: 505-872-4780
Toll Free: 888-835-5669
E-mail:kidshealth@familyvoices.org
Family Voices is an organization of families throughout the United States who have children with special health needs. The organization includes caregivers, professionals, and friends whose lives have been touched by these children and their families. The parent membership has a wealth of knowledge and experience, teaching and learning from one another. Membership is a diverse group, representing a wide variety of children, health conditions, families, and communities.

Fragile X Research Foundation (FRAXA)
www.fraxa.org
FRAXA was founded in 1994 by three parents of children with fragile X syndrome to support scientific research aimed at finding a treatment and a cure for fragile X syndrome. Fragile X research is drastically underfunded, considering its high prevalence, prospects for a cure, and the promise that this research holds for advancing understanding of other disorders like autism, Alzheimer's disease, and X-linked mental retardation. Site contains newsletters, publications, research findings and educational materials for families and physicians.

Indiana Institute on Disability and Community
www.iidc.indiana.edu/cedir/sexuality
Article by Marilyn M. Irwin, entitled *Sexuality and People with Disabilities*, includes bibliographies and referenced

materials on the topic. Links for other disability-related organizations and topics are referenced as resources. Published by The Center for Disability Information & Referral (CeDIR), the Center's mission is to provide access to information to meet individuals' disability-related needs through print, non-print, and human resources.

National Downs Syndrome Society
www.ndss.org
666 Broadway, New York, NY 10012
Telephone: 212-460-9330, 9:00 am–5:00 pm Eastern time
Toll-free: 800-221-4602
NDSS Fax: 212-979-2873
Email: info@ndss.org
Website contains subscription information for a newsletter update. Materials are available in Spanish.

National Fragile X Foundation
www.fragilex.org/home
Established in 1984, The National Fragile X Foundation stated mission is to unite the fragile X community, to enrich lives through educational and emotional support, promote public and professional awareness, and advance research toward improved treatments and a cure for fragile X syndrome. The website contains a free online newsletter, information resources for parents and physicians, links to other related organizations and topics and research. Materials are available in Spanish.

National Information Center for Children and Youth with Disabilities (NICHCY)
www.nichcy.org
P.O. Box 1492

Washington, DC 20013-1492
Phone: 202-884-8200 (V/TTY)
Toll-free: 800-695-0285 (Voice/TT)
Fax: 202-884-8441
Email: nichcy@aed.org
NICHCY is a nonprofit national information and referral
clearinghouse that responds to questions about children and
youth to age 22 (through high school) on all issues of disability. Publishes newsletters, issues briefs, fact sheets, and general
information in addition to maintaining a library and database
of additional information. All information is provided free of
charge. Services provided: database, information dissemination, referral service, resource center. Disability(s) served:
cognitive, hearing, learning, physical, speech, vision. Certain
publications are available in Spanish.

NOLO

www.nolo.org
Nolo identifies itself as the nation's leading provider of self-
help legal books, software, and web-based information and
tools. Since its founding in 1971, Nolo has been making the
law more accessible to the public.

Resource Center for Adolescent Pregnancy Prevention, Education, Training and Research

www.etr.org/recapp/research/journal2001
McCabe, Marita P. Sex Education Programs for People
with Mental Retardation, Journal Summary. October 2001.
   This summary includes the following sections: An Introduction Sexuality and Sex Education, Attitudes Toward Sexuality, Sexual Needs and Deinstitutionalization, The Need for
Sex Education, and Implications for Practice. In this review
article (published in 1993), the author looks at the state of

sexual education programs for people with developmental disabilities. The author outlines the opportunities and services needed by people with developmental disabilities.

The American Association on Mental Retardation
www.aamr.org

Since 1876, AAMR has been providing leadership in the field of mental retardation. AAMR is the oldest and largest interdisciplinary organization of professionals (and others) concerned about mental retardation and related disabilities. Over 9,500 members in the U.S. and 55 other countries have chosen AAMR as their association.

The ARC
www.thearc.org

Formerly known as the Association for Retarded Citizens, The ARC is the national organization of and for people with mental retardation and related developmental disabilities and their families. It is devoted to promoting and improving supports and services for people with mental retardation and their families. The Association also fosters research and education regarding the prevention of mental retardation in infants and young children. State chapters of The ARC may be located by visiting the website.

The Council on Exceptional Children
www.cec.sped.org
1110 North Glebe Road, Suite 300
Arlington, VA 22201-5704
Toll-free: 888-CEC-SPED
Local: 703-620-3660
TTY (text only): 866-915-5000
Fax: 703-264-9494

The Council for Exceptional Children (CEC) is the largest international professional organization dedicated to improving educational outcomes for individuals with exceptionalities, students with disabilities, and children who are gifted. This organization serves as an active advocate for improved governmental policies, establishes professional standards and provides for professional development. As an advocate for newly and historically underserved individuals with special support needs, CEC assists educators and other professionals in obtaining conditions and resources necessary for effective professional practice.

Society for the Autistically Handicapped
www.autismuk.com

Parent organization is based in Great Britain. Information covers basic assumptions about the sexuality and sexual development of young people with autism.

Trace Research and Development Center, College of Engineering
University of Wisconsin at Madison
www.trace.wisc.edu
5901 Research Park Blvd.
Madison, WI 53719
Phone: 608-263-1156; 608-263-5408 (TTY)
Fax: 608-262-8848
Email: info@trace.wisc.edu

Trace Research and Development Center is a University of Wisconsin–Madison research center that strives to design a more usable world for all. Its research, funded primarily through NIDRR and NSF, focuses on making off-the-shelf technologies like computers, the Internet, telecommunications products, and information kiosks more accessible through a process known as universal design. Services provided: database, diagnostic/evaluation, information dissemination, research center, training. Disability(s) served: cognitive, hearing, learning, physical, speech, vision.

Waisman Center

www.waisman.wisc.edu/www/mrsites

The Waisman Center is dedicated to the advancement of knowledge about human development, developmental disabilities, and neurodegenerative diseases throughout the life span. The Center is one of nine national facilities and includes a Mental Retardation Developmental Disabilities Research Center and a University Center for Excellence in Developmental Disabilities. The site includes linkages to other informational resources and organizations.

Index

Understanding Health and Sickness Series
Miriam Bloom, Ph.D., General Editor

Also in this series